The Mental Challenge of Dieting

by

Earl F. Spence, Jr.

DORRANCE PUBLISHING CO., INC.
PITTSBURGH, PENNSYLVANIA 15222

Contents

Introduction

Not another diet book. I of all people should know better than to write a book on dieting. It's funny how you lose a little weight and suddenly people think you are an expert on weight loss, health, and good eating.

In this book, I'm not telling you anything you probably do not know. This is just my experience of being hard headed and trying to lose weight my way without the expense of a weight loss center or some diet pills or programs.

The biggest and greatest battle in losing and/or controlling weight is the mental one. What the mind wants, the mind will fight to get! He who believes in oneself will win.

I'd like to thank my family, pastor, and friends who talked me into writing this book, especially my pastor who first planted the idea. Most of all I'd like to thank GOD for giving me this opportunity.

Let the game begin!

Chapter One
The Search For a Reason

The Beginning

A diet is a learning process. It's not just simply learning about food and exercise, it is also learning about one's own body. You begin to understand how your body reacts and adjusts to certain foods. The best example is how some people can handle alcohol and others cannot handle alcohol, or how some people break out when they eat seafood. The most important aspect of the learning curve is the lesson about self. If you learn this lesson, or just understand it, you will succeed. The key lesson is food dependence. It took me 14 months into my diet before this fact settled into my mind.

It is human nature to want to be happy. The mind is also looking for positive satisfaction. One of the greatest pleasures is a good meal. After a long day at work, a good meal always picks you up. How do you celebrate birthdays, anniversaries, and other special events? And lets not talk about the holidays!!!

The beginning is usually the best and easiest weight loss period. The mind is excited and the results are encouraging. The first week of any diet will be one of the best weight lost weeks. The positive result fuels the mind to keep up the process. The body is in an adjustment period. So enjoy it while it lasts! It is the calm before the storm. The game has begun.

1

The Mind, The Search For a Reason

Lets examine the basic conversation in the mind. I want to lose weight. Why? Because it will make me feel better and look good. But you look good now! Hey, I want to look better. Okay, here is what you have to do.... Well, I was just thinking out loud.

The reason for losing weight must be greater than the sacrifice of the weight loss process. The end product, the new you, has to be worth the struggle to get there. The search for a reason may take longer than the diet itself. For years upon years, I kept saying "I'm going to lose some weight". First, it starts with setting time frames without concrete start dates. Next, it was the new years' resolutions, which ends within the first month. Then finally, the prayers to lose weight.

The reason must be good enough for the long term, especially if the process is going to take longer than six months. Losing weight for a loved one is a good reason. One must be able to handle the rough times, especially if you have a disagreement or a fight with that loved one. It may cause you to lose focus and commitment to your diet. Another sound reason is because the doctor said I needed to lose weight. Doctors say this every year. Anyway, you only have to hear the speech for five minutes and you usually forget it at dinner.

A diet is no different than any other struggle in life. There are goals and objectives. There are rewards for good works and good deeds. There is punishment for bad works and bad deeds. The diet process is liken to a prison term, with good behavior (eating habits) you finish sooner. Bad behavior (cheating regularly) prolongs the process. Just remember one bad day can cost you two to three good days. You only have a limited amount of breaks (bad behavior) before the body will respond.

The reason can be liken to a war. If the army is motived and believes in the cause, they will fight without end. An army

2

lacking motivation, is an army destined to fail. It is up to the commanders in charge (The mind) to keep the army focused and motived. Keep reminding them why they are fighting and the good they are doing. Keep re-enforcing the reason for the diet. Every inch is a struggle. You may not see the result today, but tomorrow you will. The enemy in this case is the stored fat cells in the body. The extra energy the body has saved for a rainy day. Unfortunately, the sun is shinning with no rain in sight.

The diet process can be like a person in a row boat in the middle of the Atlantic Ocean. Surrounded by water, but unable to drink any. Constantly tempted to drink. It is the fresh healthy foods in your boat versus the sea of high fat, high calorie foods that taste good. The mind must be able to row to land with limited drinks from the sea. Once on land you understand that the sea can only be tamed, but not conquered. Tamed in a way that you understand the pitfalls and have the ability to ride the waves. Unconquerable, in that a little sea water is not fatal, but re-enforces why the sea must be tamed. One can enjoy a piece of a cheese cake with ice cream and whip cream from time to time, but eating it every day can cause one to gain weight.

The reason is the ultimate goal. It is the final prize. It makes the day in and day out struggle worthwhile. The ultimate reason, do it for self! Don't let self down. If self is not worth the struggle, do it for someone or something that self loves or wants more than self itself. And when all else fails, do it for GOD!

Remember you are fighting today for tomorrow. The reason, give the mind a goal, target, a cause to go on. With a good reason, the mind will fight to the end. The mind will overcome any struggle placed in the path of reaching the goal. Yes, the reason must be worth the struggle.

They have changed the name. They say that it is now weight control, weight reduction, weight management, or even a change of life style. No matter what the terminology, it is still a diet. The mind is still trying to cope with less. The new words sound nice. They add a little class, but the task is still the same. Does better packaging change the product? Is it the perception of the product that makes it work? It's the old sugar pill trick. You think the doctor is giving you medicine, but the pill is actually sugar. The mind is the actual cure, because that is where the illness is. But when the mind knows the pill is sugar, the pill does not work. So dispense with the sugar coating, if it is a diet you are on, then a diet it is.

Motivation is another of the pitfalls that can derail a diet. How many times have you decided to do something, but just could not get motived to start the task. One of the explanations is deep down you were not totally committed to action. The price was too high. One way to keep motived, is to keep your eyes on the goal, the prize. Think about what it takes to win any game. A strong start is always the best. Protect the middle, so that you do not lose any ground. Finish with desire, believe you are unbeatable.

The mind is locked into a struggle. The struggle if isolated within the mind, is a difficult one, but the outside forces are hard at work. The outside forces are admirable. Big food corporations are trying to convince you to buy their products. They feed on every sense, temptation, and reward systems. The newer ads even go after your logic(intellect). Yes, your need to be special, to reward yourself, to aid your depression, and even to enhance your sexual appeal. They tap into your memory banks, and help you visualize the smell of food. They have captured the glory days of your youth, when you could eat anything.

Flashback to yesteryear, when everything was rosier. When big was better. When doing exercise actually meant playing with your friends. Yes, enemy number 1, the food commercial.

But wait, the defense and offense of the diet has a new friend, Science. Modern science can remove or add motivation at a drop of a dime. Just watch or listen to the news. Today, they will

4

tell you that this food item is good for you. Tomorrow, there is a new study finding that this food item is not good for you. Or "do you know what's in the chicken you are eating" type of reports. Even how humane they are treating that turkey. The mind will use science to justify it's case. Just believe in the body's defense systems and take the news about science and food with common sense. Science, enemy number 2.

The third enemy is the weight management programs themselves. Please do not get me wrong, most of these programs work! It's the after part that is critical. These programs are crutches for the mind. After a while the mind becomes dependent on the program. One begins to believe that they need the program to help them lose weight or control their weight. If you are this type of person, then by all means join one of the programs. Remember these key words, the weight management programs are businesses. They are in business for profit. How much they will deviate from their program's plan for your personal needs is a big question! These programs are motivational aids also. They are trying to keep you motived to stay on your diet and in their programs. Remember the reason must come for within!

The mind is always looking for the easy way out when it comes to weight loss. It is easy to get caught up in the promises of weight management programs and exercise equipment manufactures. The end results always looks great. The course looks easy, but you only see the beginning. The hills and pot holes are different for each individual, it still must come from within, the reason, to reach the finish line. A half hour doesn't seem like a long time to ride a stationary bike, walk on a treadmill, or walk outside, but what do you do to occupy the mind during this time while the body is at work? The quick answer is to watch television or read something. Whatever the answer, it has to occupy your mind, because these types of exercises can get boring.

Are you one of those people who have tried many weight loss programs and diets? Have you tried and tried but continue to fail? Are you now complacent to the fact that you will always be overweight? Are you at the point of giving up? Why? Why has the diets and programs failed for you? Is it a matter of will power? Were you totally committed to the course of action of the program or diet? One cause for failure is that these programs are developed for the mass public. That means they have developed routines that conform to the majority of overweight people. What if your weight loss/control is an exception to the rule. The situation could be that you are following their plan, but your body takes longer to adjust. Another question, can the mind accept the restrictions placed upon it by the diet program? If the diet program requires you to drink eight - eight ounce glasses of water a day, could you? I know I can not. Second cause for failure, why are you in the program? Where you taking the advice from someone else about the program? Did the commercial or ad in the newspaper sound too impressive? Did you try other programs that did not work and figure why not try this program? In all the above questions, the reason to lose weight was defined by outside sources (loved ones, family, friends, peer pressure, an employer, or Madison Avenue) not from within your mind!

The battle of senses, the internal battle within the mind. The right side of the brain versus the left side of the brain. The wants and rewards systems versus the need system. The economists would call food a necessity and luxury good. That means to a point we need food, but at a certain income level our taste and wants for food changes. As food becomes more of a luxury good, the sight, smell, and taste of the food is more important than the nourishment. At this point the want systems begins it struggle. I want that pound cake. I want that steak. It's like a child in a toy store, in every aisle there is something. It does not matter what the last answer was, this is a new toy, a new want. We Americans, we want the latest and the greatest. The economist underlining theory is that human wants can never be satisfied. That whenever a want is satisfied a new want replaces the old want. (Just look at children when it comes to toys. As soon as they get the toy that they wanted, they see another toy that they want with equal or greater value then the last toy.) This is the case for food too. How often have you looked forward to a meal only to find yourself thinking about the next meal or dessert. Or simply eating a piece of cake only to find out that you want more cake, or piece of pie, or just something else to eat, no matter how big or small the first piece. Your need to eat is replaced by your want to eat. As one want is satisfied, another want surfaces. This is what is meant by unsatisfied wants. The only thing that stops the wants is that your stomach has no room to store the additional food, but you may still keep trying to eat. Your wants are placed on hold for a short time, then the process starts again. This may not be true for everyone or every day, but it does happen, especially during the holidays. Yes, the economist term can be related to our current situation, the need to eat versus the want to eat. Where the latter means that the body already has the food it needs for energy, but the mind wants more food. The battle, mind versus body.

The coach, the mind, must keep the players and the senses, motivated and happy. The coach must keep the players focused and on course. There are always distractions during the game that can cause the team, the body, to lose. There are the other players, people, commercials, and temptation, that are ready to take you off course, sometimes by accident. The coach must keep the players constant attention, always ready to play defense and to defend the body. The coach must also be ready to accept setbacks and use the setbacks to gain strength to continue to press on down the field. The coach must understand the game within the game. That the adjustments by the mind will be countered by the body. That sometimes you have to settle for the short gains before the long gains are available.

The reward system and friendship. How many times have friends shown you their appreciation by offering you food. How often has a friend offered you chocolates, candies, or cookies and you had to refuse them because you are on a diet? Does this make you feel guilty? This can break down your will and cause you to accept the sweets because you do not want to hurt your friend's feelings. That one piece of sweets leads to a second or third piece, and then you just blow the whole day off. At that one instance in time, the feelings of your friend is greater that your reason for the diet. Then there are the friends who will not take no for an answer when you refuse their food offering. In their defensive for you to have the food, they said that just one piece is not going to hurt you. Which may be true. If it is something that you really like, then you are more likely to give in to their request. My defense is a good offense in this case. I tell my friend that yes you are right, but you did not see the other people offering me treats. This usually gets them to withdraw their request for me to have the sweets. If you accept the sweets, one day that friend will ask you how your diet is going. You may say not to good. Then he will ask you why. Will you remember all the treats that you where offered and could not refuse? Or will you just blame the diet that you have chosen? Unless that friend has gone through a diet process, they may not understand your struggle, and everyone's struggle is different. We each have different pitfalls and weakness.

Some people say that they can lose weight any time they get ready. That may be true. But they have a problem getting ready. They can not find a reason to get ready to lose weight. Yes, some people do say they can lose weight any time they get ready. Is this something their mind has made up, or is it something to tell family and friends to get them off your back about losing weight? Do you go on a diet and lose 5 to 10 pounds then stop saying that I can lose the rest without a problem? Then you actually gain the weight back, with an extra pound or two. Yes, the first couple of pounds will be the easiest to lose. The change of eating habit catches the body off guard, but the body quickly adjusts to the fact that less food is being consumed. Is it at this point that you end your mini diet? Or did the smell of mom's apple pie drive you off course? The reason was good for the short term, but at the first sign of trouble, out went the diet. Do not kid yourself, self denial and commitment is needed. Ask how many of us Catholics complain about a day of fast or even a half day fast? But we often go the whole day without eating until dinner! See the difference, in the latter case, the mind knows it can eat at any time, that it is not being denied food, but time does not permit eating. In the first case, the mind is being told no, which increases the want of the food. Try a half day fast just once, for no other purpose but the simple denial aspect.

Remember the story when you where a child, 'The Little Engine that Could'. There is no mountain that I cannot climb as long as I believe in myself!!!

They said that there are two things you have to do in life, pay taxes and die. Some people avoid the first, but no one has avoided the second. There is also an unwritten rule that there are two things you do not argue about with people, religion and politics. Most people have already made up their mind about the two. Very rarely can someone change another persons view on the two given subjects. So too must the reason to diet come from within. The desire to change, to accept challenge must come from the soul. The reason, the minds search for the reason, must come from within. With mind and soul in togetherness, the body will follow. Very few will understand your struggle and pains. Others can offer encouragement and advise, but if the change is not wanted, then their words fall on deaf ears.

The reason is there. Will the mind bring it to the surface, or will it stay deep down in the corners of the mind, hidden! The choice is yours. The game not only began, but you are playing it without knowing the rules. The mind requires wisdom to win the battle. The search for the answer must start from within, because all the other information is available. Good Luck!!!!

Chapter Two

Diet Concepts

The Three Type of Days

The New York Knicks had a good game yesterday. The team was playing excellent defense. Their shot selection and passing was just superior. Yesterday was a day that the Knicks could do no wrong.

The New York Mets played lousy today. They had five mental errors in the field where they just misplayed the ball, this does not include the four recorded errors. The pitchers could not throw a strike, and the Mets' hitters were swinging at anything that came up to the plate.

This USA Tennis Cup match is any players match to win. Both players seem to be lost out there. Any one close play will determine the winner. A momentum changer is needed by one of the players to pull this match out.

Bob has run an interesting race today. But he just can not finish it. It is his race to win or lose. Bob must find it within himself to finish strong or he is going to lose today.

Losing weight is no different than any other struggle in life. Some days you can do no wrong, like the Knicks. Your will power is at its maximum, and no one can offer you any type of food temptation. Then there are the bad days. When you just can not handle the diet, the Mets. Your will is at a low and every other sense in the body can only think or relate to food. Then there are the in-between days, tennis and racing matches. Days when your will is down, but not out. You can fight off most food temptation, but if certain foods or drinks pass your way, you would not be able to control yourself from consuming the food or drink.

During the diet process you will have good days. It is unmistakable that you will have your bad days, especially around the holidays. It is the in-between days that one must fight for to stay in control of one's diet. The in-between days make or break a diet. If too many in-between days fall into bad days then the diet is over. The in-between days are the make it or break it of any diet. Usually it takes just one event during the day to change the status of an in-between day.

The in-between days are evenly matched opponents. The coach, the mind, is constantly in a struggle to ward off the bad influence and to keep motived on the diet. How does one fight off the **will** to cheat? Have you ever watched some of the professional players, be it basketball, football, baseball, volleyball, or tennis talking to themselves. They are constantly trying to motive themselves, to take their game to a higher level. To understand the last mistake they made and overcome it. They are searching, proving themselves, trying to think of the next winning move, or simply confirming to themselves that everything is okay. That they can handle anything that is throw their way. Yes, watch them beat on their heart and understand what they are saying; to win, it comes from within. To win you must have heart!!! The old saying goes, 'Where the heart goes, so does the mind'.

So approach the in-between days with an open mind and heart. Remember each day is different. Draw on the good days, and learn from the bad days. Rome was not built in a day, so you will not lose it in a day. Remember the lessons from Rome. It took longer to build than it did to fall!! Rome fell not from the outside, but from the inside. It will take you longer to lose weight than it takes you to gain weight.

Overview

What is a diet? Is it just a word? Is it an answer to a question? Is it a conversation piece? A diet demands courage from self. It prompts caution from others. A diet is a test of two wills. Your will for self control and your will for happiness.

A diet, a word often spoken out of need not want. A diet is a hill very few are willing to climb. From a straight line to a mountain and all in between is a diet. Its size and shape is as individual as the person who sets out to climb it.

Diet, the body's way to rid itself of unwanted / unneeded energy (fat) cells. Diet, the mind's temporary escape goat. Diet, the next subject after the weather. What is always coming but never arrives, the start date of a diet. A diet once started is always looking for a stop date.

So many people asked how to lose weight, but do not want to do what it takes to complete a diet. I have told my story so many times to my friends and co-workers that I can tell my story in my sleep. But my words have fallen on deaf ears. It reminds me about the story of the rich man asking Jesus what he has to do to be saved. When Jesus started to tell the man everything that he needed to do, he was okay until he found out he had to give away his money. So it is with my friends when they hear my story, reduce food intake, cut out the fat, and exercise. It was number one and number three that gave them the most problems. I now have reached the point that I tell them that when they are ready to start the diet to give me a call. I'm tried of hearing myself talk.

Diet, wishful thinking? Diet, I will say the word before somebody else asks me when am I going to lose some weight. A diet, it can be greater than self. A diet, its worth the gain of self improvement.

Terminology

I ask you, can new terms actually replace what has to be done? Does giving a person a new title instead of a raise in pay help that person pay the rent? Is the image or glamour more important then the financial reward? Is the title of Manger with a pay of $55,000 a year salary better that the title of Director with a pay of $45,000 a year with the same job responsibilities and authority?

Does the terms downsizing or rightsizing ease the tasks of the people that have been let go by the company? Is not the two terms the same as being laid-off? Is not the two terms, especially rightsizing, just a justification for the company's management for doing the laying off? Is weight control, weight management, or change of life style, the same old diet just with a different name?

Let not the terms fool you. The actions are the same. The approach is the same. To lose weight, one needs a reason. A reason to fight. A reason to struggle. A reason for the commitment it will take to lose weight.

Are new terms just a way to solve old problems? Do we try to solve old problems with new or different approaches? Only to find that this new or different approach applies the same principles to the problem after awhile? Are the new terms nothing more than external motivational tools? That some how, some way, we can fool the mind into believing that this is not the some old problem, that this is not a diet? It is the subconscious mind that is not motived by these new terms. It is the subconscious mind that must be satisfied by the reason to diet. It is the mind that consciously may want to diet, but subconsciously the mind does not want to

13

sacrifice anything. The subconscious is asking the question, how can I diet without giving up anything?

These questions are echoed in many problem areas. It is said internally within the mind. It is asked between spouses. A wife turns to her husband and asks, if you love me, how can you cheat on me? It is asked by the student when it comes to studying or going to a party? It is asked by the coach to get his players to practice harder and with more emotion. It is the NO word again that is echoed so many times though the mind. It is the constant 'NO' word to self about food that causes dissatisfaction, but self can justify why the answer is NO. It is NO to temptation that self has a hard time justifying. Because there is no answer. Why am I tempted by this food? It is these type of NO responses that must be overcome. It is the want of food without rationale that must be conquered. Sometimes it is out of boredom that we eat. It gives us something enjoyable to do. It is being part of a group that makes us want to eat, to share in the festivities. It is out of happiness that we eat. The joy of the moment can be savored by cheese and wine. It is out of sadness that we eat. I need something to pick up my spirits. It is out of love that we eat. Eat for me, my love. It is in death that we eat. I will eat and drink this day to celebrate the life of my friend, who I will not forget.

Be it temptation or emotions, we sometimes eat for the wrong purpose. This eating will not be replaced but it can be controlled. It is the controlling of the temptation and emotional eating that the subconscious must accept. Whatever thoughts are in the subconscious mind, most of the time become active thoughts in the conscious mind. It is in the conscious mind where they are acted out. Question, is impulsive buying nothing more than the subconscious mind taking control of the conscious mind? It is after you made the purchase that you wonder why you purchased that item? The answer never really comes to you clearly, but you are satisfied with that answer. You say to yourself, 'why did I buy this anyway?'. Then later you say to yourself, 'yes, okay.' without any further questioning or justification. The answer was always within you, it just was not at a conscious level. So too must be the reason to diet, it must encompass the whole mind, the subconscious and conscious mind, or there will be troubled waters ahead. If the mind cannot answer the 'Why' question when it comes to a diet, the diet is in trouble.

Words of Encouragement?

The words echo within the walls of my mind. How much did you lose? How did you do it? Please explain to me what I must do to lose weight. What can I say to the person that does not have the will to lose weight? What words can I say to you to convince you to pick up the cross, and begin the process on getting the new you, the you that only you dream about?

The modern world calls it weight control, weight management. Their words are true if one is at the weight one wants or should be at. How can the term weight control refer to me when I am seventy pounds overweight? Weight management, what does this term really mean? What management style do I use? What techniques are effective for me? The terminology has added a little class to a dull and ugly word, diet.

An even greater terminology used now is that one does not diet, one must change their life and their approach to food. This statement is true, but I disagree in that what one needs to eat when one is overweight will be different when one reaches their goal weight.

A diet is not just a matter of changing ones eating habits for a time period to compensate for extra energy the body has stored for future consumption. A diet is a struggle. It is a struggle to unlearn bad habits. It is a struggle to temporarily change ones food rewards and stress management systems. It is a struggle between wills, happiness versus necessity. Where the price of happiness is extra weight. Its a struggle of mind versus body. Where both need

15

to survive. Where the mind knows the body and what the body needs, but does not understand the body and how it works. Modern science is still trying to answer this question. One day, we will be able to conquer the common cold.

A diet is a NO signal to the mind. NO, you can not have that cake. NO, you can not have the second helping of food. How often can you say NO to yourself? The internal struggle is like a child and a parent. The child is also testing the parent to see what they can and can not get away with. A child's search for information is constant. Why mommy? Why daddy? Can I have this? Can I have that? The child begins to wear on the parent. At some point the parent either breaks down or pushes the child away. The smart parent understands the child's game and plays with the child. Answering the child's questions of why. Posing questions to the child. Asking the child, why do you want that? Testing the child, 'Is that what you really want?'. The struggle of parenthood, it never ends.

The NO answer to a child is done out of love. It is for your own good, the parent tells the child. The child only understands NO. It is not until later in life that the child understands what the parent meant by NO. It is then that the child appreciates what the parent has done for them. It is then that a deeper bond between the parent and the child is developed. So too is the struggle within the mind. When you start a diet and began to cheat or wonder why you are on a diet, you must start to play the role of the parent. Understanding that some of your wants are simple wants. Sometimes we want just to want. It is the act of eating that you want not the food itself. Self denial is the key. Can the will of self, control the child within self? There is a child within all of us. Search for the answer to the questions; 'why I want to eat'. Some of us find the answer and pass the test. Others find the answer and do not believe the answer, so they fail the test. Still others find the answer and are too scared to work though the answer, and fail the test. Then the last group simply do not take the test.

16

Some people are good parents by nature. Other have to work hard at being good parents. Just like some people can eat anything they want and not gain weight. While the most of us must watch what we eat. During the diet process, the strong willed, will have an easier time then those of us whose wills are not as strong. The reason for dieting makes the difference. It gives the will something to fight for.

As one begins to think about going on a diet, what enters the mind? Is there a moment of sadness? I guess that depends on how much weight one has to lose. Is there a moment of denial, disbelief? I can not be this heavy. Is there a moment of hopelessness? I have tried this diet program and that diet program but I still can not lose any weight. I stand before you like a teacher trying to teach a difficult and important subject to a class. The teacher ponders, what can I say to the class to get the class motived? What words can I use to explain the importance of the subject? What words can I use to give you the knowledge of the subject? What can I say that will make you want to learn? Have all my words fallen on deaf ears? Is it I who have failed you or have you failed yourself? Is it my fault, the diet program, that I did not give you all the knowledge needed to pass? Did you try your best to pass? Did you do the homework as assigned? These questions go unanswered. Every unsuccessful diet must address these questions.

A diet, it is me versus the program. The diet program, has the developer gone though the program? Do the developers know what they have asked of me to complete their program. So many questions, so few answers. The reason must come from within!!!

The diet programs offer education. They try to teach you the ins and outs of food. What to look for, what not to look for within the food groups. But do they truly understand the struggle to lose weight? Are their words of encouragement from the heart or is their motive to keep you in their program? Can I tell this person my true problems without them being recorded in some journal? Do they truly understand my problem? Diet programs, can I afford the cost of the program? The diet program, did I get the full story in the beginning?

A coach echoes a challenge to his players. So powerful were his words, that the players went out and played the best game of their careers. A good coach understands his players. The coach knows when to give a pat on the back. When to give a harsh word or two. Most of all a good coach is a good listener. It is he who listens that gains wisdom! It is in the stillness that one begins to understand the lesson. It is at the library one seeks the wisdom of books and the stillness to comprehend the words. So too is the search for a reason. A quick answer is usually a wrong answer. He who speaks without first listening to his body, speaks without knowledge. Are the parts of the body greater than the whole? Is the mind greater than the body? Each has a role to play in self. Does not the heart pump blood to the brain? Does not the brain tell the heart to pump blood? Does the heart have to suffer a heart attack before the mind accepts that it can not overeat? Are we so set in our ways that we disregard the warnings as false alarms? Does not history tell us anything? Every major struggle had a warning signal? Can not the Africa animals tell when danger is near? Does the Zebra wait until the Lion is within striking distance before it tries to make its getaway? Is it not too late at that point for escape?

Does the yellow light mean stop or go? Is it not a caution signal? It is at this point one has to make a choice, stop or go. Choose wrong and you may receive a ticket or be in an accident. But the majority of the time you will get away without any problems. It just takes one time to guess wrong and actually have to pay the price. Then we think its unfair, but were we not warned of the danger?

Dieting is like investing in the stock market. You have to be in it for the longer term to really see any gains in your investment. Unfortunately, some people are quick to take a short

18

term profit and pull down the value of the stock, which in turn leads to a longer period for the stock to fully maximize its value. One should avoid cheating just because one received good results. It is these temporary setbacks that causes a diets to fail, just because, the next week you usually do not lose as much weight. Dieting is all in the mind!

I offer you these words, it is not until the reason is worth the struggle that one will really begin to diet. The answer to the question of why I must go on a diet must come from within because you are the only one doing the fighting, the hand to hand battle is within self.

Chapter Three
Emotions

DCD

We are human beings. By nature we need to be rewarded for a job well done. We also need a relief outlet for the times we are down or depressed about something. Depending on your motivation factor and length of period for your diet, you will need a break from the diet process; a vacation. If you are not a workaholic, then you will need to look forward to something different or special.

Please understand, one of the hardest things to do is to get back on a diet program once you have gone off for a meal or two. It is just like work, after a vacation the first day back is always the hardest.

If I can use work as a comparison, the diet and cheating aspects are like work and vacations. After an extended period of work, one looks forward to a vacation or a day off. The things that sometimes keeps one going is the vision of one's vacation and the fun that will be had on this vacation. So too is the diet process. After awhile, one would like to have a piece of cake, pie, fried food, or whatever is not allowed during the diet. Its the simple fact that one cannot keep telling the mind 'NO'. With this in mind, I developed DCD, which stands for Designed Cheat Days. This is where a day or a meal on a perceptual day I set aside to cheat on my diet or for a better use of words, have a vacation from the diet.

These DCD's help me to get over the ho hum days. The simple fact of knowing in three weeks I was going to allow myself some special meal was enough to get me through the current situation (problem). DCD's came about through the need for change, something different. As one begins to restrict certain foods and drinks, the mind has a way of looking upon those items as rewards. DCD's can be shared days. Days set aside when you are going out with friends or family and you do not want the restraints of the diet holding you back from totally enjoying yourself.

As you move along in the diet process the DCD's began to become spaced out more. Instead of every two weeks, it moves to every three weeks. The mind begins to deploy more energy to ending the diet then its need for rewards or satisfaction. One begins to watch what one eats. All of a sudden, the cheating is not as bad as it was before. Actually, the cheating may just be adding a little variety to your diet.

DCD's are the vacations away from the diet, even if its just a brief moment. DCD's are like visitors visiting a prisoner in prison. It breaks up the monotony of the day. Yes, the mind needs something different, sometimes a YES answer instead of a NO answer. Remember you are being hit day in and day out by food, sometimes you must slip a step to spring forward.

In the beginning the DCD's will pose a challenge. The challenge is going back on the diet process after the meal or day off. After a couple of times, the transfer will get easier. If you find you cannot handle going back on the diet after the DCD, change what you are eating on the DCD or just give them up.

You will find that once the mind knows that a DCD is coming, it will prepare the body for that day. A couple of days

21

before you will notice that you are eating just a little bit less or you have increased you exercise. The mind and body may not always be on the same page, but they tend to work together.

DCD's have a down side. The down side I find to be is that if the meal is not what you expected, you feel like you have cheated for nothing. This can lead to planning another DCD sooner then you wanted. So whenever at all possible, keep your expectations in check.

DCD's, temporary relief from the battle of the diet.

Cheating (Good versus Bad)

What do you consider cheating? Is it anything that is not on your diet? Is it simply overeating on any given day? What does cheating on your diet mean? It may not be your fault that you cheat on any given day. If your boss decides to take you out to lunch, do you refuse because you are on a diet? Or do you take your lunch along? This may be a condition out of your control, but what can change into a meal of cheating is how you handle the situation. Do you figure hey, this does not happen often so I will enjoy myself and throw my diet to the wind for this meal? Or do you do the sensible thing and eat a low calorie meal? A lot of people figure that any meal out should be held as special and that the restraints of the diet should not hamper their happiness. This may have to do with monetary value more than anything else. Some feel it is a waste to spend money on a meal that you can not enjoy.

Cheating simply mean a diversion from your diet program. For an example, if you are on a weight maintenance program that requires you to purchase their food, you may want a break from their food. So you decide to eat something different for dinner. You go to a supermarket to buy a Budget Dinner that is low in fat and calories. This is cheating in the sense of the word, but it should not be considered cheating. This is good cheating. It is a need for a change of taste. The taste buds just needed to be refreshed.

In the above example, cheating is bad if the low fat, low calorie dinner is replaced with hamburgers or a thick steak. Even though this is bad, sometimes it is necessary to carry the dieter over the long haul. That is why I created the DCD's stated earlier. The bad cheating can cause one to derail a diet. It can also cause one to postpone a diet that is in progress. The bad cheating is caused mostly by the sense of taste. When this sense is satisfied, it gives great pleasure to the mind. In the moments of disappointment and anguish, the sense of taste can stimulate the mind with great satisfaction, and bring calm back to the mind.

Cheating is also a matter of control. Control in controlling one's appetite. I know that peanuts are high in calories and fat. But the fat in peanuts are the good type of fat. I also know that any diet should contain some nuts. So I like to enjoy cashews from time to time. My problem is that if I buy a bag of cashews, which is eight ounces, I can not stop myself from eating the whole bag. I consider eating the whole bag cheating. Even though the cashews are good for me, eating the whole bag is not good for me. It is this control aspect that I consider cheating on my diet. What I needed to defeat this problem was to find a smaller bag of cashews. But like most people now days, the small bag did not give the economical value of the larger bag, thus some of the appeal to cashews was removed. My greater sense of value outweigh my willingness to cheat.

What must be done in any struggle is to find a higher purpose to help you overcome the current difficulties. Cheating good or bad must also be related to your reason. As stated before, sometimes a small setback is good for the overall diet. At some point you may find that the things that cause you to cheat can not be solved by the food you have chosen. This will be explained in more detail later in 'Understanding Self'.

Some good cheating may need to be included in your regular diet program. I found out that the greater the choice for foods available, the easier for the mind to handle the diet. Some people are very creative when it comes to preparing foods. You should keep this creativity when experimenting with food, but not with the high fat foods. With the changing times there are a lot of foods and spices that are available in low fat and salt free. The reduced salt helps keep the water weight out of the body.

Cheating good or bad, it's the mind's search for relief. Once again the reason for dieting can help contain the need to cheat. The weaker the reason, the greater the temptation to cheat. The stronger the reason, the less cheating needed. The search for a reason encompasses many things and many avenues of the mind. Cheating is an extension of the reward system.

The Shark Effect (The Eating Frenzy)

If you are like me, then you tend to eat not because you are hungry, but because food is available. Are you one of those people who buys a bag of cookies and just cannot put the bag down until the cookies are finished? Can you leave a small piece of cake for the next day?

After a period on my diet I was sitting in front of the television watching one of the nature shows about Sharks. I watched as the divers put chucks of fish in the ocean to attract the sharks attention. When the first shark arrived on the scene, it surveyed the food for a few minutes. Then when it deemed it safe, it began to eat. It would take a bite, then swim around. Take another bite and swim again. By the fourth or fifth bite other sharks had arrived on the scene. Then it was simple mayhem. Anything in the area that looked eatable the sharks ate without first examining the danger. The sharks even attacked the divers in a steel cage.

I began to think. Sometimes when I eat it was the same as the sharks. Once I started eating, look out. Eating for nutrition was out of the question, the animal instincts took over. It was not enough until the prey was no more. The words Left - Over meant the crumbs that fell to the floor. And once the prey, food, was gone, the search for more food was under way. Yes, just like the sharks, I attacked the food. I know I'm not alone with this approach to eating.

Now that I recognized this Shark effect, how do I remove it. Once you recognized this need to eat massively from time to time, it may not be captured, but it can be tamed. I used two approaches to handle this. The first approach was I combined my lunch with dinner. This allowed me to eat the same amount of food as normal, but it feed the mental need to eat a large portion. Another way I handle this, was to eat large salads. I know, salads. This is what I put in my salad, lettuce, tomatoes, cucumbers, boiled chicken breast (2 - 3 pieces), and 1/2 - whole honeydew or cantaloupe. With the fruit and chicken, it did not seem like a salad. It was more like dinner in a bowl. The honeydew/cantaloupe give the chicken a different flavor. The lettuce helped give the large portion. In this way the body was happy because of the nutritional value of the meal, and the mind was happy because of the amount of food consumed.

The Shark effect may not be of your own doing. Some foods can trigger this emotion. Especially snack foods that are light in weight but heavy in calories. Corn chips, potato chips, and pretzels are just a few of the examples. Even some of the foods that are good for you can lead you astray. Peanuts are high in fat. It is good fat, but even too many of them can derail a diet.

Madison Avenue has know about the Shark effect. Just examine some of the commercials for food products out on the market. Even the sizes of the French fries have increased. Is it the concept of giving you more for your money or just the concept of feeding the Shark effect! There was even a commercial that said, 'I bet you can't eat just one.' Every commercial for food products will have to be judged on its own merit. Just like every one will have to judge what causes them to act like a Shark.

The Shark effect can also be an approach to a given situation. How many people just can not leave any food on the table. Have you gone out to dinner with a friend and that friend could not finish their meal. What made it worse was that the friend did not want a doggie bag. Did you find yourself reaching into your friends plate to finish off their meal? Some people do not like to see food go to waste. Here is an another situation. You or someone in your house cooks a big meal expecting friends and family to come over. But a few people do not show up and since the food doesn't taste as good left over, do you find yourself eating just a little bit more? Do you keep picking in the pots? Do you feel compelled to eat because the food tastes good or because it took so long to cook, or simply because it is there?

The Shark effect is not just limited to food, but drinking also has this effect. Alcohol and soda (regular) can lead to the shark attack. This is more than likely to happen in the summer when more liquids are needed. Alcohol, as they say is empty calories. Which means the calories in the alcohol drink gives the body no nutritional value. Soda is high in sugar, and its the sugar that makes you want to drink more.

I noticed my Shark like behavior sitting in front of the television. This is just one of the habits I had to break. But after further review, I noticed what was causing this Shark effect, boredom. Sitting in front of the television I needed something to do that was enjoyable. Something to go along with watching television. Eat food was the perfect answer. So as I watched television I wanted something to eat. Potato chips, peanuts, fruit, it just did not matter. At one point the combination was so great that I wouldn't eat my lunch or dinner when there wasn't anything good on television. The combination had a third element that I had to break first, I also had to be sitting on the couch, lazy boy chair, or even worse sitting on the bed, to maximize enjoyment. The major problem with this was that I would fall asleep after I finished eating. Thus, I broke one of the unwritten rules, don't eat before going to bed. Now that I knew one of my problems, I had to find a solution. The first step was to stop eating on the couch, chair, or bed and eat at the dinner table. This was a major step. By enforcing this rule some of the excitement was gone. I still would watch television, but the dinner chair is not a place where I can fall asleep. Thus it forces me to get up and do something. Still sitting on the couch while watching television can cause the mind to want food. I solve this by drinking coffee or tea. I think it was the action of doing something while watching television on the couch that I had to conquer. The coffee or tea helped me get that full feeling and since tea and coffee are calorie free, it was no harm. Except running to the bathroom every now and then. The only draw back is what you put in your tea or coffee. For my tea, I put a sugar substitute, zero calories. In the coffee I put skim milk, this helped me get the daily amount of milk one needs. Besides, I just can not drink milk by itself. This problem, if I play by my new rules, is solved.

As I began writing about my shark effect on the couch, a thought of how did all this come about began to ponder within my mind. Then a possible answer flash, baby. One of the first senses a baby trusts is the sense of taste. Everything that is new must be tasted. If the item tastes good, then it is eaten. Any bad tasting items are quickly disregarded. Is it the baby's search for understanding or the need to be satisfied that cause them to put everything in their month? The baby uses the only sense it can understand, taste.

Taste can be taken a step further, whenever a cop needs to know whether an item is a drug or poison, they have the tendency to place a small amount of the item in their mouth to taste it. The sense of taste and enjoyment can lead to the Shark effect.

So the waters out there are rough and deep. Keep your eyes open and your senses keen, and you will conquer all situations. Remember there is a Shark in all of us.

The Reward System

The good will be rewarded. The bad will be punished. We have been told this every moment of our lives. We hear it at church, at home, at school, and at work. The ultimate reward is heaven. The ultimate punishment is hell. The reward systems have many levels. Just like in school, the passing grades are from A - D, with a D meaning you just passed. There is only one failing grade F. It does not matter what range you fall in, you just fail. There is no border line. No gray area. The F covers all the failing range from zero, those who do not try, to 59, those who just failed. But failure today does not mean failure tomorrow! Learn from the bad, the pitfalls, to help you improve the good.

This is the typical reward and punishment system. During a diet process, one must examine one's reward system. There are two aspects that need to be reviewed. First, how do I reward myself for good weeks and good results from the diet? Second, how do I reward myself in general?

From time to time one will want to reward oneself for good performance on their diet. The best question is how do I do the rewarding? Each person's values are different. Some people may buy themselves some clothes. Others may purchase a piece of jewelry. Then there are the others like me, who would buy a nice meal. If you are like me, then you have a problem. How can I satisfy my need to reward myself and also my need to stay under control on my diet? Here again your reason has a big impact on the type of reward you select. In my case, the reward was simply a DCD. I combined my need to cheat on the diet with the need for a reward. As the diet process moved forward, I needed less and less rewards. Good results became common place, so the need to reward the results lost their importance. Also the reward itself was my ability to keep to the diet. If you can, build rewards into the diet process.

This step is not easy! This is where many diets are won and lost. One cause is that the mind starts looking for rewards. It is like cheating is a reward. Rewards are great in the beginning. Choose a reward base and stick to it. Set goals, but not in concrete. Reward the goals that are met, hopefully without food. Learn from the missed goals. An example of a missed goal is setting a weight reduction of ten pounds for a month. At the end of the month, you only lost seven pounds. The cause could be easily explained. One, the ten pounds was unrealistic. Second, your body has adjusted to your diet. Third, not only did you lose seven pounds, but you lost an inch off your waist. The latter should not be considered a missed goal because your body adjusted the weight reduction.

Rewards and DCD's can work together. If you have food rewards, choose one or two dishes that you really enjoy. Set those two aside as the ultimate reward. This is the reward that you will only enjoy when you reach your diet goal. This will give you added strength during the diet process and add a little extra flavor at the goal setting day.

Remember rewards are tools for the mind. Some people will not need rewards during their weight loss process, others will. Please keep in mind the reason for going on the diet and that will be a reward in itself. Rewards are reduced over time for good behavior. As it is written in the bible, why do you want a reward for what you are supposed to do? This relates to the diet process in that as you understand yourself more and more, you are supposed to adhere to your diet because you have the understanding of what it takes to succeed. Do not become a trained Seal act, always expecting a piece of fish for every trick performed!

Rewards are part of life. How does one reward oneself? A lady purchases a very expensive dress. When she begins to ponder the cost, she simply says, I deserve this dress because... The purchase is no longer filled with guilt, it is now a reward. A parent tells their son, since you did so well on your report card, I'm going to buy you that computer game, Street Fighter, you wanted. A husband who sees his wife working hard at work says; hi honey, you been working so hard lately, I brought you a cheese cake, and it's your favorite flavor, strawberry. After a hard day at the office, one may reward themselves by going out to have a couple of drinks with some co-worker. This is especially true. Or some may say; hey, I feel good today, I'm going out to dinner.

Rewards from yourself and from others are hard to handle during a diet process. Not because they are not nice, needed, or wanted, but because food rewards tend to throw a diet off course. How can one reward themselves for a good day at work? How can you reward yourself for accomplishing something special (closing a big deal at work, purchasing your first home or car, improving your golf score, or selecting the right stock)? If the reward is going to be a nice dinner at a nice restaurant, then do not go overboard. A lot of people think that this is only one night so why not do it up special and forget about the diet. If you have been doing well on your diet, then this may be okay. But remember the old saying, pay me now or pay me later, but you are going to pay me. Which means that if you did not prepare before the meal, you will have to work after the meal. If you have been on the borderline with your diet then, you may have a week of disappointing weight lost results. This can lead to frustration and a weakening of your will power. In this state, the mind is more apt to cheat. The NO word to food can not be handled by the mind as well as before. The reason for the diet will start to be questioned. You will start to think that it is impossible to lose the weight you want. In the worse case, you may start to look at yourself as a failure. Do not let your reward system hold you back. The weight loss is worth the struggle, keep the faith in yourself. Replace or rebuild your reward system. It is a change that may need to be done. But where there is a will, there is a way. The process continues, the search for a reason will encompass many things. A reward is not a reward if guilt is associated with the reward. It's like receiving a stolen coat for Christmas. If you know the coat is stolen, can you really enjoy the coat?

Stress

What is your threshold for pain? What is your threshold for pressure? What is your threshold for stress? What is your stress release mechanism? What is your tension release mechanism? Just like rewards there are stress and tension releases. Like the reward system, when the mind is troubled it looks for comfort. Some people reach for a drink of alcohol. Others look for the relief in drugs. Still few take the healthy way out by exercising, working off the tension. That leaves the rest of us that reach for food.

Your relief system is second nature. When we reach that threshold, our relief systems just kicks in to protect the mind from a total breakdown. Once we have found something satisfactory to ease or remove our stress, we will stick with the relief item, be it alcohol, drugs, exercise, or food. We are creatures of habit. Most of us were born into habits. School, work, and play all fall into schedules. Anything that changes that schedule is met with resistance. We like the safety of the schedule. We are so afraid of change sometimes that we stay in bad situations even when something better is offered to us. There is a saying that I do not agree with, the devil you know is better than the devil you do not know. I say if you can not handle the devil you know, how much worse could you be with the devil you do not know. There are angels out there to help you along your new path. It is also a learning process about self.

This is not about stress management. This is simply to inform you of some of the hidden pitfalls that can derail your diet. These are the troubles and problems that only you know. The old saying I need a drink of alcohol because... It is the relief, or the belief of relief, that the alcohol gives that takes the mind to a more relaxed state. That one may start to think or talk about whatever is troubling them. Whether or not this solves anything depends on any given situation. Some of the problems with alcohol relief is that it can lead one out of control of self and trigger false hunger pains. This lead to overeating and depressed weight reductions during that week. The unfortunate part is that one mostly will not remember the overeating.

Those of us who seek stress relief from food have a different conflict. The need of relief versus the control of the diet. Most of the time the food that one consumes on the diet is not what gives relief from stress. It is usually our reward or cheating food items that relieves our stress. What would you rather have, a carrot or carrot cake? The carrot probably adds fuel to your current fire. In that one may sink to a lower level because one can not get relief, and this time it is self denying the comfort that makes it harder.

I to had to wrestle with this problem. I was driving home one day and I was upset. I wanted a bag of potato chips. The more I wanted the potato chips the more I knew I should not have them. The internal conflict was reaching a feverish pitch. Just then, I realized that the potato chips were not going to solve my problem. My problem was still going to be there in the morning. In fact, I knew when I finished the potato chips that I was going to want more food. I also knew the guilt that was going to be associated with the potato chips. At this point, I realized that the potato chips were not going to solve my problem and I went about trying to solve the problem without the temporary relief of the potato chips.

Stress management does not always mean relief. Some people like to eat when they are stressed to help them think, to clear the air. It is in this relaxed state that their mind is free to think. Evaluation can now be performed on the current troubles and/or problems. It is like taking a glass of warm milk at bed time to help you sleep. It is like your mother hugging you when you where a child, and she would tell you that everything will be all right. Just these calm words were enough to give you peace of mind.

There is one more stress that you may face. It is the stress of the diet. The diet itself can be stressful, simply because it is a constant conflict within your mind. How much does it take to control your eating habits? How often can you say NO to yourself? Are your weight loss results what you excepted? These questions have different answers. The day you ask yourself this question you may be in total control of your diet. How will you handle the stress of the diet? The answer is always within self. Do not punish the body for the mind's need for a break. Dream, yes dream of something fun. Something that takes your mind away from food and the diet. The best thing you can do is keep busy. Give the mind something else to think about. Get a mind teaser game. Find an outside distraction. When all else fails, go to sleep. The diet may decrease your stress threshold. It may be an underlying pain in the neck. Face the facts that bother you about your diet. Find a way to adjust the diet to suit your personality. Remember 'package' diets do not work for everyone. They could cause you to hate the whole diet process.

There is no easy answer to stress management. An ounce of prevention is a pound worth of cure. This is something to think about before you start your diet. Stress days may just be a bad diet day. Just write it off and move on with your diet. But unless you can remove what is causing you your stress, then you are in for a long hard fight with your diet. The outside pressures will cause more and more desire for relief. Another way will need to be developed to handle the stress if the diet is going to succeed. This stress eating may prolong the diet by reducing your weekly weight loss, which in turn will prolong your time on the diet. This in time can lead to dissatisfaction with the whole diet process.

Stress management is a subject in itself. I am not trying to offer you any answer on how to deal with your stress. Stress is just another one of life's elements that you will have to confront while you are on a diet. A prolonged period of stress or unhappiness can have adverse effects on your diet. This is another cause as to why diets fail.

Stress and the diet, do not overlook the relationship! Good luck and stay stress free!!!

Depression

Depression has just settled in for a moment during this diet period. One wants to slip back into the old self, the old relief systems. It is time to look to the refrigerator for relief. Something nice, something good, something to remove the troubles. But wait, the mind wants to fight on, to stay on course for the diet. Internal conflict, mind versus mind. Relief systems versus the reason to diet. Today the reason wins the battle. Internal damage has been done. The person is not happy. Do you face your problems or sit and mope? Today will be forgotten in the near future. All signs of struggles and conflicts from this day will be gone, only the results from the diet will be available. It is the next depression that one must prepare to conquer. The reason must stand supreme. The will power of self must be greater than self's relief system. The struggle of dieting is a mental one. Depression, anger, sadness, stress, happiness, pleasure, joy, and rewards are the emotional outlets of the soul. What is a normal day? Are you content about your current situation? Depression asks the question; 'Why me?', 'What have I done wrong?'. The diet sends depression one level deeper. Self searches for relief, it finds the reason to diet. It does not help the depression, but it calms the mind. Can you cope? The diet must continue. The reason must be good enough to handle the full spectrum of emotions. The diet will end one day, but what depresses you will always be there. The diet process may help you overcome many things, hopefully depression relief. It is not easy to lose weight. It takes patience, it takes time, it takes will power, it takes a reason. See you at the finish line.

Chapter Four
Special Events

The Holidays

The birds are singing. The children are laughing. There is excitement in the air. There is something special about the holidays. Whether it be summer or winter, spring, or fall, each holiday brings it own joy. Christmas and Thanksgiving are the most thankful of all holidays.

Holidays offer a challenge to the one who is on a diet. Holidays also represent food, special foods. Pies and cakes that mothers and grandmothers only make at the holidays. It is a festive time, when the old English saying comes to mind, "Eat, Drink and be Merry". It is a time of remembrance of the past. It is a time to remember all the loved ones and friends who can not be there with us. It is a time of joy!!! Food and presents are how we show that joy. Yes, the holidays and food, a combination that is hard to separate.

The ideal goal during the holidays is to lose weight during that week, even if it is less then normal. The more common approach is to stay even, just maintain your current weight during that week. And of course, the last thing we want to do is gain weight. Your goal should be not to gain any more than a normal weekly reduction. That is, if you usually lose 3 pounds a week, then you do not want to gain any more than 3 pounds. The ideal mind set is to maintain and enjoy the holidays, not gain and regret the day after.

Now the big question, how does the mind handle the holidays. It is best if you treat the holidays as DCD's. That is, allow the mind to prepare the body for the up coming events. The holidays will no doubt be harder then a DCD, but the approach is the same. First, there is the pre-holiday mental preparation. That should include increased exercise, reduce intake at dinner, or elimination of desserts. The preparation period or duration really depends on how much you plan to deviate from your diet. With this in mind, you can plan your meals and you will be more aware of overeating. Next, the day of the holiday, you should do some form of exercise before the meal. Something simple like, a 30 minute walk, a slow jog, some jumping jacks, or ride a bike. This will help burn some extra calories and reduce the impact the meal will have on you. It also comforts the mind in that it takes away the guilt of eating off your normal diet plan. You may not feel guilt today, but tomorrow you will, especially if you are not progressing with your weight loss as you would like. At the end of the day of the holiday, try to do some very light exercises, to go to bed on a positive note. Exercises like, jumping jacks, walking or jogging in place, or a few sit-ups. This way you will feel that you have earned that meal. It will add more joy and excitement to your day. Lastly, the post holiday period is simply getting back on your diet as fast as you can. The only way to remove the guilt is to remove the weight.

The approach to the holidays is different for Christmas. Only because the Christmas holiday can extend over a period of days, depending on your work environment.

What is it about the holidays that causes us to release all controls that we have about controlling our weight? What does the mind tell the will to justify the additional food intake? Why is it that to really celebrate a holiday we must eat? Hundreds of years ago that's all they had. When family and friends came over they stayed for awhile. It took days to cook that meal. Taking celebrating back to the beginning of this country, Indians shared the meal with the new settlers. The enjoyment of settling down with new friends and family to share some of the graces given from GOD. So it has become a tradition to celebrate with food in this country, not with just food, but with a feast. And depending on your nationality the feast can have many courses before the main meal. How do you stop Aunt Sally from piling the food on your plate? How do you stop Uncle Steve from telling you to eat, get in the spirit of Christmas? How do you handle the complements from your sister, Emelda, saying 'you look good, you can afford to skip one day.'? Yet will you remember these words two week from now when the diet has stalled? What will you say when your co-worker says, hey I thought you were on a diet? Remember in the end, the reason must come from within. If you plan to take the holidays off of your diet or an extended DCD, prepare for the after affect. Remember, it's not the earthquake that always does all the damage. It is the after shocks that can cause more damage than the earthquake. The after shocks are working on a weaker foundation. A bridge standing on one beam does not need much of a shift in the earth to cause that one beam to fall. It is the same with the dieter, once the day is lost to overeating, one thinks that another piece can not do any more harm. It is that piece, after shocks, that causes the diet, the bridge, to fail. Think about it!!! Enjoy your holiday, the spirit of the holiday.

Everyone talks about the Christmas and Thanksgiving overeating. The news shows are full of advice from the experts about what foods to watch out for. The Christmas overeating usually starts at the office parties. Lunches with your boss and/or co-workers. Then there are the after work get togethers with close friends to celebrate Christmas. Yes, the Christmas feast starts weeks before Christmas day. Then there is Thanksgiving. This is one of the biggest feasts of the year, if not the biggest feast. Where the big spread is placed upon the table and the food is piled high on the plates. And to top the dinner off, there are the desserts that make your mouth water. Best of all or worst of all, depending on your point of view, there is food left over for days. If you are among the group that get Friday off, then the feast does not stop. Thanksgiving, a time of joy, remembrance, celebration, and food. The food preparation for Thanksgiving starts days in advance. Some of the dishes take a day or longer to prepare. Grandmothers and mothers have to start cooking early because there is not enough time Wednesday or Thursday morning to cook all the food. Its the scene of smell that incites the mind. The kitchen oven is working overtime. Food, that is all the mind thinks about, the food it cannot have. Yet it is not that you should not have the food, but only in moderation.

Let's not forget the other holidays that are celebrated with picnics. Memorial day, Fourth of July, and Labor day. Hamburgers, franks, sausages, and chickens are on the grill. Add dad's special barbecue sauce and it makes for a fun food day of eating. Are you the active type? Do you get out and play any volleyball, baseball, softball, or touch football? Or do you sit around playing cards and talking? How can I forget about the beer and wine. Yes, what is a picnic without the beer. Do you feel out of place if you do not eat or drink? What is a celebration without eating? Or do you figure the exercise will more than compensate for the extra food you are eating. The problem is that one piece will not harm you, but can you stop at one? Can you once again stop your aunt or uncle from filling up your plate. Question, if you eat before playing any sports, will you be very active in the sports if you play? What is the answer to this question of eating at picnics. It depends on your reason. Your reason is your justification, defense, and comforter. It is why you should not have the extra piece of barbecue hamburger. It is the defense that you tell your aunt and uncle to stop them from piling the food on your plate. It is the comfort of knowing that you did the right thing. Remember if you do not tell them you are on a diet, then when they deem it time for you to eat more they have more force to push the food on you. Because without telling them you are trying to cut back, your defensive line is weak.

There are three mind sets for the dieter. Depending on how much you believe in your reason, you fall into one of these situations. One, I'm not going to let any diet spoil my holiday. I'm going to enjoy myself and worry about the diet later. Second, I'm going to stick with my diet, but I will eat only the food that is within my cheat border. No rich food and no apple pie, sweet potato pie, or cakes. I will not slip during this week. Third, and last group will not give in to the holidays. They will enjoy the diet meal even while everyone around them feasts on the meal. Where do you fit in? The second dieter I think is the best. Just because the dieter has the ability to adjust the diet to given situations and challenges. This will enable the dieter to handle other situations that pose the same threat as holidays when it comes to food.

Eating Out

It's the holiday season. A couple of co-workers and I decided to go out to lunch, it's their idea, to celebrate the season. The big question is upon us, where to eat. The three of us are on diets. But I'm the only one totally committed to the diet, for I have found my reason.

Once seated at the restaurant and menu in hand, I began to ponder the choice of foods. I'm looking for the lowest calorie food with the least amount of fat. You see, eating out poses a challenge, a challenge of self control. I glance over to the ladies and I see that they have lost it. There is no dieting this meal. The dessert word has been spoken already. My choice is simple, I'll have the salmon, boiled with no butter. I stress to the waiter the word PLAIN, no butter. Why add the extra calories. My taste sense has adjusted to the diet. Anything to drink, the waiter replies. Yes, a cup of hot tea is my response. The ladies reply, you are sticking to your diet. I only smile.

The ladies in turn order an appetizer, onion soup with the cheese along with their lunch entrée. When they are asked about a beverage, they responded with soda.

What a tale of two different sides of dieting. For me, I began to think about making up for this meal. Even though the food was on my diet, fish and the rice that comes along with it, I still was not sure about how it was prepared. Would they still put some butter on my fish? Is there any butter in the rice? After a moment or two, I was back into the conversion.

Needless to say, the ladies did order their desserts along with coffee. I just join along for coffee. It may be only one meal, but it is the self control that is important to me. Besides, that would mean at least one more meal under the diet.

So I ask you, what is it about eating out? What makes eating out so special? Eating out is fun, it is a celebration. A diet is dull, it is a struggle. A diet is not a happy time. No one ever smiles when they say, 'I'm on a diet'. It is a sad word. Eating out is a reward. After completing a project at work, my manager wanted to take me and another co-worker out for lunch. To reward us for a job well done. At first thought, one would jump for joy, but I just looked at it as another test. Another struggle to stay under control. The choice of restaurant was a Chinese restaurant. This was okay, especially since this time I was the only one on a diet. My selection of food this time was the steamed mixed vegetables with steamed rice. This time I was sure I was getting plain food. My only concern was if I was going to have to reduce my starches that night. Always thinking about making adjustments for eating out. My lunch partners had no problem with what I had ordered, since they knew I was on a diet. They actually admired my ability to stick to my diet. This of course did not stop them from ordering what they wanted to eat.

Again I ask what is it about eating out that challenges one's diet? Is it the fact that we see eating out as a reward? Is it the fact that if I want to eat healthy I should eat at home? What is more enjoyable about eating out, the food, the company, or the atmosphere? Do you eat out to experience different foods? Do we eat out just to be in the company of a loved one? Do we eat out to be part of the in crowd? Do we eat out because we do not want to cook? All are valid rationalizations.

Think about children for a moment. Do you see the joy in a child's eye when you tell them we are going out for dinner? Do you see the excitement when you tell them that we are going to McDonald's? Is McDonald's hamburgers any better than ours? Is it the excitement of the trip that lights up the child's face? Is it the fact that they know that they won't have to eat any vegetables that is joyful? What is it that is so exciting about eating out for children? Remember, there is a child in all of us. Does eating out bring back the good days from childhood? Look within yourself for the answer.

Some of the appeal to eating out is that you usually eat foods that are too time consuming to cook at home. The dishes that take hours to prepare and minutes to eat. Eating out is simply about food. The title says it all, Eating Out. Eating out also allows one to be adventurous. Adventurous in that one can try foods from other nationalities. Being on a diet limits the adventurous in us. It takes some of the fun out of the food. The diet is now a business. It is profits and loss. What the mind profits, the body loses.

Eating out when you are on a diet takes courage. Courage in that one needs to be able to handle any negative feedback from the waiter or your dinner partners. Courage in the understanding that you are only limiting one aspect of eating out, the food aspect. The good company and atmosphere are still there. The food does not take away from the conversation. What is the difference between eating a piece of boiled fish and fried fish? Only the calories. Is the way the fish is prepared going to take away the mood of the evening? Only if you let it. Will your dinner partner stop talking to you because you are eating fish and not steak?

41

Eating out does not have to be a signal for a vacation from your diet! Look at some of the other elements of eating out that are pleasant to you. Limiting your food intake does not mean the end of life. A diet is about adjustments. Both mental and physical. You are unaware of the adjustments the body makes, but the mental adjustments are what causes a diet to fail. As in business, the business that does not adjust to changes is out of business. In the animal kingdom, if the animal does not adjust to natural changes, then it is extinct. Just look at the dinosaur. Like man, the country that does not adjust is left behind, and in the old days conquered. A diet is about change, be it short term or long term.

Eating out, it is not a signal to cheat. Eating out has some built in guilt. Be it monetary or emotional. Be it a reward or stress management. Eating out must be addressed before, during, and after the diet process. Adjustments must be made to satisfy, both mind and body.

Eating out on the special days, mother's day, father's day, birthdays, and other celebrations. How does one handle taking mom or dad out for dinner on their special day? Do you skip this day because you are on a diet? I'm sorry mom but I'm on a diet so that means I can not go out to dinner with you. The responses will vary with different mothers, but you will not be on the top of their list. These are events that you have to attend. Either you control the dinner or the evening will control you. The best avenue is to eat light. Choose foods that are low in calories and fat. If you must join in the toast, try the non-alcohol drinks, light beers, juice, or soda. This way you are part of the celebration and holding true to your diet. Your mother or father will appreciate your company and admire your will power for your diet. If this approach is not for you, then treat this special day as a DCD. This way you will have mentally prepared for this day already and surprisingly you will be more under control because you have set your limits within your mind.

Eating out, the challenge between dieting and happiness. Eating out is only a challenge because of the values that have been associated with dining in a restaurant. If a restaurant cuts back on their portion, then the customer would be upset. Eating out and dieting is a contradiction in most peoples minds. No matter how you are doing on a diet, whenever you go out to a restaurant to eat with family or friends they expect you to stop dieting for this one meal. I do not know why this is true, but true it is. Do not let outside forces try to control your diet. Once these outside sources find a way to break you down, they will do it more often. You are like a boxer who can not take a left punch to the jaw. Once your opponent sees this weakness, they will always be trying to throw that left. Show no weakness when it comes to your diet and eating out. Explain if you can that you have to work off this meal. Tell your friend or family member how special they are that you have given up your diet for one meal to share a moment of joy with them. Let it be know that from this moment forward you are back on your diet. Defend your diet process. Show how determined you are to complete the process. The only true way to show progress and determination is to show results. You are like a report card, you only show a grade, pass or fail. No one sees the work you had to do to get that grade. You will be judged by others only by your grade, not how hard you tried. The only person you have to show a passing grade to is yourself.

Eating out, it can be controlled and fun at the same time. Eating out, a dieters test. Good luck and take heart.

Fun, Food, and Drink

It's party time! Fun, food, and drink, it's the nightmare of the dieter. How can I diet and have fun, are the sentiments of the dieter. Is it the setting that causes us to eat at parties? Is it the host that causes us to eat at parties? Is it the toasting of the event that causes us to drink at parties? Is it the mood of the party that causes us to eat and drink? It is the same old question, how can I say no thank you without offending? How can I be happy without a drink in my hand? How can I be happy when I rather be indulging in the feast? Parties are temptations to the dieter. No matter if one can fight the temptation to eat or drink at a party, the party still has a negative impact on the mind. The mind has said no to itself, that means at some point it must say yes to itself. Its the simple justification to oneself, see I was good at the party, I deserve a reward. Nothing changes, how often can you say no to yourself? The more you can, the better off your diet.

Wedding, birthday parties, card parties, baby showers, bachelor parties, bridal showers, baptism, and the party list goes on, they lead one to question one's reason to diet. The self denial and self determination needed at parties is greater than normal. Your emotional need to be happy and to celebrate is greater at parties. To be part of the party group and not a party wall flower. Your memories of past parties and the good times that were had, play havoc on you. Can you sit at a table and watch other people eat around you? Can you sit at the table and handle the smell of the food? Can you constantly repel the request to have something to eat? Can your mind handle the situation? Can the reason to diet justify the need to be good? The reason to diet versus the fun, food, and drink. The battle is within the mind. It is civil war. If the mind wins, then there is new and greater self and determination to the diet process. If the mind looses, then the diet process has been extended for a couple of days/weeks. Too many mental losses and the diet is over!

All hope is not lost. One must have a plan when it comes to parties. A couple of things that you can do before going to a party; one, eat before the party that way you will not be tempted as much. Second, do some exercise before and after the party. Third, treat the party as a DCD. Fourth, try to stay away from the people who give you the greatest temptation to eat or drink. You know yourself the best, what causes you to cheat and what gives you strength. It is the pleasure sense that makes parties difficult. It is not just the pleasure that parties give, but the activities that are associated with the party. It has become the unwritten rule that at most parties there must be alcohol. It is only recently that you start to see alcohol free parties. The better parties offer food. It's not that offering food is bad, but the foods usually offered are high in fat and calories. It is these negative jolts to the body that causes the dieter problems. Once again, it depends on how good you have been on your diet that determines the true effect. No matter what the effect on the body, if it places the mind in a negative state, then that is trouble. Trouble in that it starts to weaken one's will power.

To have fun at a party one must be flexible. One must be able to select items, be it food or drink, that can fit within one's diet plan. To be able to satisfy both self and party host. To eat, but only a small portion. For example, if the party host is serving fried chicken at the party, accept one piece of chicken. Select the smallest piece available. Also remove the skin off the chicken before eating the chicken. By removing the skin, not only do you remove calories, but you are removing fat calories. If they have salad at the party, fill you plate with more salad than other food items. This can hide the food you are not having and the salad is good for you. Besides, with a plate in your hand they will not bother you to eat. Most times it does not matter what you eat, but that you did eat at parties. If its drinks that you must partake in, then chose the drinks that are lowest in calories, like light beers. If mixed drinks are more your taste, use more water or juice in the drink. Also drink slower than normal. Savor the drink like fine wine. Don't get into the mind set of losing the day to cheating. This can cause you to go overboard. You will find yourself drinking or eating more than you normally would. This is because internally you feel that you will not be able to do this type of eating and drinking again. You justify to yourself that its only one day and it will not hurt. But it is these types of events the leads one astray. Its like the alcoholic saying just one drink will not hurt. You know yourself. Do not put yourself into situations that you can not handle. The key is moderation. With moderation the body can withstand these one time jolts to the diet.

45

Dieting is not fun. Partying is fun. Its like oil and water, the two do not mix. It is this internal mix that must be found. The successful dieter learns how to adapt to life challenges. A party offers the same problems as holidays and eating out. These events do not change or decrease the need for self satisfaction. Events outside your control only make your need to satisfy yourself even greater. Dieting by nature is a depressing state. One likes the positive results of dieting, but not the process it takes to receive those results. Dieting means giving up something. It means self denial. When food and drink is part of the fun, it brings guilt to the diet process. The guilt can be conscious or subconscious, but it is there. Only positive results (weight loss) can remove the guilt. Guilt lessens the motivation, which question the reason, which opens the doubt. Dieting is not fun. One has to re-learn how to have fun while dieting. This temporary change in one's habits is the key. One can not postpone life while one is on a diet. Dieting requires adjustments. Like a child who lost their favorite toy, that child quickly learns to play with another toy. The same is true with dieting, you have to adjust your life until the diet is over. Who knows, maybe the other toy was better than the lost toy!

Fun can be had while on a diet. Partying is okay. One just has to change one's definition of having fun for a short time. Fun, food, and drink, a combination that is hard to beat. Enjoy life and fear not. Have a plan and you will have fun while dieting. Maybe not to the degree before dieting, but fun never the less. The game within the game.

Chapter Five
Dieting and Food

Food Pleases The Attitude

Eating is a necessity for life. Dieting is unlike smoking in that it is harder to diet then to quit smoking. Simply because you have to eat. Some of the smokers out there may disagree with me but that's okay. I do not have the experience first hand of trying to quit smoking. I have heard this sentiment spoken from others who have quit smoking and have tried or are trying to diet. Food pleases the attitude. Good food engulfs the mind with excitement and joy. Food turns a bad day to a bearable day. An average day to a good day, and a good day to a great day. Food can calm what ails the body.

To me a good dinner puts a cap on the day. No matter what type of day it was, dinner always makes it bearable. The day ends on a good note. Yes, food pleases the senses. Food calms the mind.

Food, a stress manager, brings pleasure to a bad situation. Food, the item of celebration. There is no problem with food being a stress manager or a motivation tool. Food must be controlled by the mind. The dependence of food in any given situation must be reviewed. Is food just another way to handle the problems at hand? Some people try to drink their problems away. The pleasure that food brings must be examined with great detail. If the reason for the diet is not strong enough to control the pleasure of food, then the diet is in trouble. In trouble in that the need for relief is greater than the need to diet. The longer the problem or situation, the longer the diet can be derailed. This could lead to the termination of the diet. For example, when I was young and on a diet, I could not resist potato tots. Whenever they where served in school for lunch, I would eat lunch otherwise I would skip lunch. I make up for the potato tots in other ways by reducing what I ate for dinner or doing some more exercises. This is a case in point that a weakness for a food must be overcome during the diet process if the diet is going to be successful. The potato tots was not a stress relief but a joy to the mind. The joy that the potato tots gave me was greater than my desire to lose weight. But to receive this joy, I had to give up other foods to counter balance my joy and keep my diet on track. It is a give and take relationship. To gain greater joy for certain food items, you have to give up food items that give you lesser joy to the point when they neutralize the impact on the body.

Food is enjoyment. I do not know what is greater, the joy of eating or the food itself. Mostly a combination of both. There is something about sitting down and eating a big meal. There is excitement in the air. Where do I start, what item do I eat first? No matter how full you are, there is some sadness when you come to the end of the plate. You just want one more piece, especially if that last piece was the best tasting. Even if you do not want a second helping, there is something about a full stomach. Something pleasing and relaxing. It is the feeling of accomplishment. This accomplishment is really at dinner. Breakfast does not give the same satisfaction. Maybe because you know you have a days work ahead of you and you know you can not relax. Lunch is the same as breakfast when it comes to enjoyment. You usually are at work when lunch time rolls around. There is always that time restriction that puts a hurry on lunch. Also a big lunch means you would like to sleep at work. Big lunches lead to laziness.

What is it about food that pleases the mind? Does it go back to the beginning of man when man had to hunt for food? Imagine what joy it must have been for the caveman to catch or kill his meal. To be able to feed his family. Is it that satisfaction that has carried forward? Maybe it is that food can not disappoint you? A good meal does not give a wrong answer. A good meal tells you what you want to hear. A good meal reassures the mind that everything will be all right. A good meal eases the tension. A good meal brings contentment when all else fails. Food occupies the mind with joy. There is nothing worse than bad food. It can turn joy sour. There is nothing like a good cook. What is the best way to catch a man, though his stomach.

Remember, food is like everything else in this world, moderation. One must learn their body. What can and can not the body handle. Too much rest, exercise, food, or alcohol is not good for the body. Food is a pleasure, but too much pleasure is no good!!! Food, energy for the body, do not overfill the tank. Food pleases the attitude, can you afford the happiness?

One must recognize what is happening before a solution can be found. Examine how food effects you and plan your diet accordingly. Whatever you decide, keep an open mind. See you at the finish line!

Starvation Diets

The mind in its haste to speed up the diet process will look to starvation dieting as an answer. It seems so easy, I'll speed up the process by not eating. This is a no no. Every doctor will tell you this fact. Every diet program will also repeat this fact. But this still holds no merit with you and the same was true with me. It is not until you have the facts in your hand that you can finally accept the fact that starvation diets are no good.

The first thing is to define my view of starvation dieting. Any diet that greatly reduces the amount of food available for consumption, I would consider a starvation diet, not just not eating anything for a couple of days. For example, eating only two slices of toast a day for your meals, I would consider a starvation diet. Simply because the body is not getting the minimum requirements to sustain itself.

During my course of dieting, I veered on to the starvation avenue to help speed up my weight loss. After a couple of weeks, the weight loss was not what I expected it would be. For all the extra struggling I was going through, I was losing only three pounds a week, my normal weight loss was between two and three pounds a week. Then one day I asked myself, why don't people who went on hunger strikes lose that much weight. You would hear that John Public is on a hunger strike to fight against the mistreatment of prisoners. The news would report that Mr. Public has now been on this hunger strike for one month and has lose ten pounds. I do not know about you, but I figured he will lose more than ten pounds in one month. As I pondered this situation, I came across an article that was explaining how the body uses fat cells and muscle cells. In this article it went on to explain that the body once deprived of food after a certain period of time will not consume fat cells but will consume protein cells. In this way the body saves the fat cells for the last line of defense. When you are to weak to move and do anything, then the body would use this reserve of energy. So the starvation dieting is actually counterproductive. One may lose weight but it is not the weight one wants to lose. Starvation diets cause you to lose muscle cells and not fat cells.

Another side effect to starvation diets is that the body's defensive systems will take over the next time you eat. Remember that the body will want to prepare for the next starvation dieting by storing extra energy (fat cells). The body is always trying to counter anything negative that the mind does. This is something that you must be aware of if you tend to add a starvation period during your dieting process. This is one of the mini struggles within the diet process, finding the right amount to eat at the same time maximizing weight loss.

Something I learned about starvation dieting is that it made me mentally weaker. Not mentally weaker in the sense that I could not think or solve problems. I became light headed from time to time during this starvation period. It was like the brain was not getting enough oxygen. My mind was more vulnerable to negative thoughts. Things that I would not normally think about started to pop into my mind. My mental defensives were at a weakened state. The mind during this starvation period passed the majority of the energy to the body so that the body could survive. I think this is why the body is so defensive. What good is the brain if the body does not survive? The body's defensive mechanism will push the mind to eat. Once a satisfactory level of nutriment is consumed by the body, normal mental functions will return.

I do believe starvation diets test your morale character to some degree. In a way that you will never do anything that is morally wrong to you, but if it is your mind holding you back from doing something, then you are more likely to do the task once weakened by the starvation diet. Case in point, some people will steal food if they are very hungry, while others will find other legal ways to acquire food. In the latter case they believe stealing is morally wrong and simply would not steal. While in the first case these people feel that their need to eat out weights the crime of stealing. Different case in point, some people say that alcohol makes one tell the truth. Once someone has reached their limit of consuming alcohol, their mental defensive controls are no longer in top form. They say and do things that they normally would not do or would normally hold back from expressing. Internal frustration now starts to surface, because there is nothing to hold back these emotions. Every one probably knows someone that once they start drinking, that person has a different personality. Starvation diets can have the same effect on the mind as alcohol but effecting a different area of the brain. Remember during a starvation diet period, the mind is constantly saying NO to itself about food. Just think about it for a moment, how many things have you done in a weakened state of mind? Only later to regret the decision that you made. We act differently, when we are happy than we do when we are sad or depressed. Starvation dieting puts one into a depressive state.

As a side note, God may have put Jesus in the desert for forty days and forty nights without food and water because God knows the importance of food to one's mental well being. It was after the forty days and forty nights that Jesus was more vulnerable to the temptation to sin because of the body's need for food and water. It was in this weakened mental state that his moral fiber and duties toward his father could be supremely tested. This was also a test that we could relate to with ease. In the end, it was more important for Jesus to obey his father's will than to satisfy his body's need for food and water. Remember the first temptation for Jesus was to satisfy his hunger.

Depriving the body of food also reduces one's energy level. The body needs the fuel from food to stay active. During the starvation dieting period, one will require more rest and relaxation. It is at this point that you will be sleeping longer and more reluctant to get up in the morning because your energy level will be greatly reduced. For awhile you will be wondering why you are tired. You will fail to put the fact that the starvation dieting is causing the problem. One other explanation is that to handle this period of starvation dieting, you have put this fact to the back of your mind. Also if you are eating just a little bit of food, you may not put the correlation between being tired and eating together because you figure that you are eating. But the food being consumed is not enough nourishment for the body, so the body is being drained of its available energy. With a low energy level, starvation dieting effects your body's defensive mechanism to fight off germs and sickness. The body is more susceptible to colds and the flu. Changes in weather conditions can also cause problems during this period because the body does not have the resource to adjust to adverse conditions. Everything the body does, it needs energy to accomplish. It takes energy to sleep. If the body does not have its energy needs replenished regularly, then it will save whatever energy it has available. Since during this starvation period the body does not know when it's next nourishment will be, it consumes what energy it has wisely. By resting and sleeping longer, it conserves energy.

Starvation dieting plays havoc on the mind and body. In the struggle to lose weight quickly, starvation dieting will throw the body and mind into an irregular state. Increasing one's stress level and reducing one's mental capacity. Before starting on a starvation diet, please beware of the pitfalls to mind and body. The results that one expects from starvation dieting may not be the results achieved. Can you handle the negative results? The easiest answer is not always the right answer! Whatever you decide, good luck.

Food and/or Exercise

What can I say about food and dieting that has not already been said? The facts are all there for you about eating. Reduce your food intake, cut out the fat in your foods, and you will lose weight. What the doctors and nutritionist said is true. The mind knows it is true, but it is the execution that is the problem. Non fat foods are diet foods to you. Diet foods have an after taste, an excellent example is diet sodas, some soda products state that there is no funny after taste because they know that has been a problem in the past. Partly because the manufactures have not invested much money into developing their diet products since there has been a small audience for the diet products. Thus, there has been no real need to improve the taste of the diet food products until recently.

Now that I have said that, here is another conflict within the mind when it comes to dieting, non-fat foods versus taste, smell, and sight. If the food does not taste good, you just will not eat the food. Well, if you do eat the food, you probably will not order that food or cook that dish again. If the food does not smell good, you are more unwilling to eat the food. Even if the food tastes okay, the next time you are confronted by this dish, you will think twice about eating the food. Third, if the food does not look appealing, you are likely to by pass it. So, some diet foods offends the three senses, taste, smell, and sight. It is these senses that must be overcome, especially taste. The key to eating healthy as they call it, is to change one's taste buds. The problem with fatty foods is that they taste good. They add flavor to the food. Fried foods just taste different than boiled or baked foods. Some food items just taste better fried. But as your taste buds adjust to the less fatty foods, you will be better off on your diet. As the facts are stated, reduce your food intake, reduce your salt intake, and try to stay away from fried foods and butters. The frying of food and butter are quickly stored by the body as fat. These fat cells are the among the last energy source the body uses. Thus it adds this fat to the reserve of fat the body already has stored. The rationale for the salt reduction is to help reduce the fluids in the body. Salt keeps extra water in the body. Water translates into weight.

Food is the key to life. A Healthy diet can add years to one's life span. But healthy foods are not for everyone. No matter how good salads may be for you, some of us just can not eat them. A dieter is trying to find the right mix between healthy foods and fatty foods. The mix is all mental. I know many friends who want to lose weight, but they can not give up fried foods. Fried chicken, fried shrimp, and French fries are just a few of their weakness. It is this unwillingness or inability to change eating habits for a temporary time period that causes them not to diet or to have their diet fail. But it is these same friends that get upset with themselves when they look in the mirror. Their mind set is that food is not to be eaten for life, food is to be eaten for enjoyment. You must find some form of enjoyment in your diet food. The mind must be happy or satisfied with the choice of foods to be eaten. In my case, I still like to eat large portions of food at my meals. I had to solve

54

this problem if my diet was going to be successful. What I found was fruit. The more the merrier. The melon class of fruits was the answer, honeydew, cantaloupe, and watermelons, especially watermelons. With watermelon I could eat a large portion and get that satisfying feeling without all the calories. The added benefit of the melons was that it gave me the water my body needed without drinking water. The key point I'm trying to stress is that my reason for my diet pressed me to search for an answer to my problem about food. I found a healthy food that I liked to replace the fatty food which I also like with the same level of satisfaction. This did not stop the craving for the fatty foods, but it offers an acceptable way to satisfy myself. In time, the craving for fatty foods decreased. The longer one stays away from fatty food, the easier for one's taste buds to change.

By reducing your fat intake you don't have to reduce your food intake as much. For example, one slice of butter is one hundred calories, all fat. That same slice of butter could be replaced with an apple which is only eighty calories on the average. I'm not saying that you should start to count calories, but you should be aware of your options when it comes to foods. Case in point, a twelve ounce can of regular soda contains 140 calories and a twelve ounce can of diet soda contains zero calories. The only difference is the sugar in the regular soda. This leads me to another point, be careful about all the non fat food items that are on the market now. A lot of them are high in sugar, which still gives the food the high calories count. What the manufacture does to make most of the food item fat free is change from regular milk to skim milk. We get so wrapped up into the non fat aspect that we fail to look at the other ingredients that can give a dieter problems.

What is the right amount of daily calories for you depends on your daily activities and life style. Your natural size and body frame can dictate how many calories you need to eat daily. Only your doctor or a health specialist can really set a detailed diet for you. But if you are like me, you can not listen to the professionals because they did not address the mental needs of the diet. What I did was take a calorie count that was generally accepted by the medical/nutritional industry and used that as my daily target. In the beginning I used 1800 calories as my daily target. With 1800 calories I receives enough food/nutriment for my body, and was able to lose weight. As my weight reduced, I moved my daily calories down to 1500. I have known some people to have tried 1200 or 1000 calories daily. The way I counted my calories was by reading the label on the food products. One must also add calories for any other items that are added during or after the cooking process. Since I boiled my food, I did not need to add any calories. But for example, if you are preparing fresh greens and add a little olive oil to the pan, then you have to add the calories for the olive oil. Or if you are baking a piece of fish and add butter and lemon for flavor, then you must add the calories for the butter and the lemon. Any health store, book store, and some supermarkets carry books on the calories of the different foods. You do not have to go to that level, but be truthful to yourself about the amount of food you are eating and how it is prepared. Whatever you do it must be mentally and physically acceptable. If the mind does not like the food or program, you will not follow the program or eat the food. If the body is not getting enough nutriment, then it will start to break down and cause you to cheat or quit your diet.

Exercise is another way to lose weight. But what exercise do you do? Do you have time to do all the exercises that are needed to help you lose weight? Can you do this exercise at home or do you have to go to a health club (gym, there is a new term for everything.)? Exercise is great when it is an active sport. Playing basketball, football, tennis, golf, or softball is great fun and a good workout. Unfortunately, one does not get to play these sports as often as one would like. If you are like I used to be (overweight by 100 + pounds), the body cannot handle the active sports without feeling the pains for the next couple of days, especially the knees. It is these pains that push you away from exercising. Exercising is also boring. It is the dullness that also push many people away from exercising.

It is the motions that the body needs to keep fit. Just like a fine sports car that constantly needs to be tuned to keep it in top shape, so must the body. Without maintenance, the sports car starts to lose performance until it runs no more. So to will the body fall to sickness and weakened health if it is not kept active. Maintenance on the sports car extends the cars useful life. Exercising increases the body's natural defense systems.

Exercise is nothing more than doing something to keep the body active. As we move from a blue collar to a white collar society, the need to exercise is even greater. The energy that we use to burn off at work is no longer being done. What makes this fact even more important is that we have not changed our eating habits. Exercise for your heart, to keep the blood pumping. Exercise for the body's defense system, to keep the body strong to fight off germs. Exercise to tone and strengthen the muscles. Exercise for energy, extra energy. Most of all exercise to burn fat.

What is the right exercises for you? That must come from within the mind. The exercise that you choose must satisfy the mind and body. One will not do an exercise if one does not see any progress from the exercise or one can not physically or mentally handle the exercise. What good are jumping jacks if your knees can not handle the strain? Can you walk on a treadmill for half a hour if the mind is too bored during that half a hour? How many people who have a treadmill or exercise bike would rather sit and watch television for half a hour than ride the exercise bike or treadmill for that same half hour? There is something about exercise that bores the mind. Even if the mind could be occupied by something else, it tends to still not want to do the exercise. Is it the restraint placed on the mind during that half hour? Knowing that during this half hour you can not do anything else that is not within arms reach of the bike or treadmill cause the problem? Maybe doing nothing is better than doing an exercise that is boring? You must find out what is holding you back from exercising. Be it finding the right exercise, or just varying your exercises from workout to workout, but find some exercise that you can perform.

A good exercise program starts off slow. Allow the body and the mind time to adjust to the new routines. Contact your doctor before you start any exercise program. This way you can be sure that your body can handle any exercises you are going to perform. If at all possible, choose exercises that you can do at home. This way you are not in any rush to get to and leave the gym. I am not talking about muscle building exercises. I'm talking about basic exercise to get the heart moving. There are a lot of exercise programs on television. You can either follow along with their program or do what I did, take bits and pieces of exercises from different programs and perform the exercises at your own pace and work on your problem areas.

For me, I started my exercise program by walking a half an hour at lunch. After I ate my lunch, I would go out for a walk. I did not do any speed walking or set any distance that I wanted to walk. I only set a time limit of at least thirty minutes. This way I had constant movement. I walked as fast as my energy level would allow. The days that I was tired, I would walk slower. The days that I had a high energy level, I would pick up my pace during my walk. What I noticed was the more I walked, the faster my pace. Once I started to get the extra energy from the walking, I decided to do some extra exercises. I had an exercise bike in my apartment which was collecting dust. I decided to start riding it every other day for at least fifteen minutes. So now I was walking at lunch and riding an exercise bike every other night. As I was riding the bike, I started to read the newspaper or a comic book. This took most of the boredom away from the exercise. Slowly I increased my time on the bike to a minimum of thirty minutes six days a week. If I did not have anything to read, I would watch television. Also, what I did was put the things I would need next to the bike so I could reach them. This included the television remote controller, telephone, the newspaper or comic books, and anything else I may have needed. This way I was mentally and physically prepared for the exercise.

Since I was going to have to lose a lot of weight, I knew I was going to have to tone my body. So I purchased a set of dumbbells to perform weight exercises for my upper body. I started by doing simple arm curls. The arm curls helped my arms and chest muscles. As a side note, since I was losing weight, I was also losing strength. I needed to replace this lost strength by developing my arms and chest muscles. One day I noticed one of the muscle exercise programs on television. They were showing various upper body exercises with the dumbbells. Since they looked easy to do, I added a few of them to my exercise program. I performed weigh exercises every other day. This is the routine that I follow even now. The exercises with weights take about ten minutes a day.

I did not want to join a health club or gym because I wanted to do something at home. The time I would have to spend going to and from the gym would have been longer then the exercise routine. Also, there would be no way to make sure that the equipment would be available when I wanted to use them. This way, at home, I was not in a rush to start exercising. It was a more relaxing feeling. I did not need any added pressure from my exercise program, the diet was hard enough.

Now the question is food, exercise, or both. Your diet should contain both, well balanced meals and a regular exercise routine. I think you should start your diet by reducing your food intake. Get the motivation from the diet to exercise. In the beginning I started to exercise to speed up my weight loss process. Do not exercise to eat more food. I feel if you start the exercise first, it may be harder to reduce your food intake because the mind feels it is already suffering with the exercising. Exercising takes motivation, especially during a diet. One must be motived to do the exercises. It is so easy to say I am too tired today, I'll do the exercise tomorrow. Do not fall into that trap. Tomorrow always comes with another excuse. Dieting or exercising take commit and self denial. There is always something better to eat than your diet meal. There is something better to do than ride that exercise bike or walk on that treadmill. The American couch potato, overweight and under exercised.

The diet, eat healthy and exercise, for the mind and body. The reason to diet, is it good enough to include exercising? The search for a reason must examine many avenues of the mind. Commitment, dedication, desire, and self denial are tools the dieter needs. Reduce food intake and/or exercise are the means. The game is within the mind! Play it to win. The struggle is upon you, it is a game you can not quit. As they said in the old west, choose your weapon (food, exercise, or both) and come out fighting!!!

Fruit, Fruit, & more Fruit

A new medical survey states that you should eat five servings of fruit a day. Long before this survey came out many people where eating lots of fruit daily. Over the past couple of years, juice machines have become common place in many homes. Juice machines help increase the level of vitamins and minerals the body receives in one serving. Many people have combined many different fruits together to get the nutritional values and taste that they have wanted.

Fruit is healthy and good for the body. Most fruits are low in calories and fat. The body can burn off the calories from fruits much easier than some of the others foods, like pasta. Fruits are great for snacks. Fruits are even great for desserts. Fruits are also good for dinner. There are fruits that can give you energy. There are fruits that help colds and flu. There are fruits that taste sweet. There are fruit that taste sour. Some fruits are higher in calories than other fruits. There are fruits for every one of the body's needs. You can add fruits to your salads. You can have fruit salads. You can include fruits as part of your dinner. Fruit, the multi purpose food.

Fruit offers the dieter a sociological benefit. This is one of the healthy foods that can replace fatty foods. It was fruits that helped me overcome my need to eat large portions. Yes, eating a whole honeydew had less calories then eating one bagel. Not only less calories, but it was also more filling. Grant it that one does need a minimum amount of starches each day, but one should know how to improvise to ensure the success of one's diet. It was something about a nice sweet cantaloupe that pleases the mind. Adding fruit to other non fat food items just makes the meal a little easier to handle. Fruit and sugar free Jell-O just taste good together. It is amazing what you can eat when the mind has a reason to diet.

Eating fruit for dinner is an alternative from time to time. It is low in calories and helps the body cleanse itself. Fruit fast days are great too. They really help the body. And depending on the fruit you chose, you still can eat a good amount. For example, on a fruit fast day you can have a couple of bananas, an apple, an orange, a cantaloupe, a honeydew, and quarter of a whole watermelon and still have a satisfying feeling of eating without all the calories. The day after a fruit fast your body will have started the cleansing process and you will feel mentally good.

Fruit may not be for everyone. If you need to switch to more vegetables, then by all means do. It will take time to overcome the need to eat large portions if that is your problem. The mind must search for solutions to whatever problem one may encounter in one's diet. Fruit is an excellent substitute for fatty foods. Take heart, it is a struggle to lose weight on many fronts. Fruit is an ally. Fruit for a snack. Fruit for lunch. Fruit for dinner. It is a healthy choice. See you at the finish line, I'll be the one with a slice of watermelon in my hand.

Chapter Six
Diet Milestones

100 + Pounds

What is it about being 100 plus pounds overweight? What does it take to lose 100 plus pounds? It takes commitment! First, lose the defeatist attitude. One must be in a positive state of mind. Second, break down the goal weight lost into target areas. For example, my first target area was to lose twenty-five pounds. The next target was to reach three hundred pounds. You can create target goals at whatever interval you see fit. I never used dates as target goals. The only time I used dates was for DCD. Build some type of rewards for reaching the target goals. Be it clothes or in my case a DCD. Third, keep an open mind. Always accept what is. Try to understand what is working in your diet and what is not working for your diet. Fourth, do not try to conquer everything in one day. This can only lead to burn out and frustration. Any runner will always pace themselves. Always saving their best for the last leg of the race. Fifth, one hundred plus pounds is a lot. Do not look at the whole number. Try to break down the weight loss into mini diets. Try to bring fun into the diet program. Use your target weight lose goals as the mini diets. So as you reach one of your target goals it will be a completed diet. This may give you the pleasure of reaching your goal and the psychological view of a successful diet. The mind must keep the mind happy, even if it is just small victories. Remember if you do not win any battles, how can you win the war? It is the victories in the battles that keep the army motived to press on with the struggles of war. Sixth, keep focus on your reason. The reason why you are dieting. When the reason comes from within, the mind will be more focused and you will learn more about yourself. Since the diet will be over an extend period of time, you will encounter many hurdles that must be overcome with different answers. It is these hurdles that teaches one about self. Seventh, try not to set any dates. Setting dates can lead to disappointment if they are not accomplished. It is the psychology of failure.

The mini diet within the diet approach is that many changes will have to be made during the diet process. It is these struggles that you should be considering your mini diets. What you do to lose the first ten pounds may be different then what it takes to lose the forty to fifty pounds. Not only may the mind set be different, the body may have made three to four adjustments and the struggle of dieting may start to take hold. Life on the diet is now the norm. The other pressures and pleasures of life start to bear down upon you. The way you normally handle these situation may be affected by your diet. It is these little things that can cause one to lose concentration on the diet, thus causing a slip in the diet, and if one is not careful, stopping the diet. Sometimes the situation leads back to old habits and one gains back the weight that was lost.

At one hundred plus pounds overweight, one believes one can not lose the weight. It is this negative mind set that leads to failed diet attempts. It is at this point one begins to look for miracle diet programs. The promise of magic diet pills and approaches that only lead to failure gives one a sense of hopelessness. I even began to look at the advertisement of stomach stapling to lose weight. Yes, their words of 'the only effective way to lose 100 pounds is stomach stapling', hipped my disbelief in myself. I began to tell my family that I have tried to lose weight, but I can not seem to lose any weight. That I will always be fat. It is this defeatist attitude that causes my diets to fail. It is not until I found a reason to diet that I truly began to lose weight. Once the reason was in place, failure was out of the question. Failure was not acceptable. Still I find it hard to give you the words that will help you start your journey to lose weight. You know what it takes to lose weight. You have doctors ready to assist you. You have weight maintenance programs ready to teach you their technique on losing weight. You have diet products ready to aid you with your weight loss. You have exercise equipment manufacturers with every type of equipment needed to help you lose weight. But it is the old saying, you can lead a horse to water, but you can not make him drink. The reason to diet must come from within. The mind once it found a reason, will find the best program to lose weight. All the diet programs or exercise equipment in the world will not help you lose weight if you are not motived to lose weight. These program may give you temporary motivation, but fail to motivate you over the long haul. Their motivational tactics only work in the short run because they only want you to buy their products. So as the mind gets accustom to their motivational tactics, the programs do not have the same effect. Or you find that the promise of the program is not what they said it would be. Thus you began to lose faith in their program, and then you end their program.

Like any other medical problem, one must face the fact that they have a problem. The road to recovery only begins once one has accepted the fact that one has a problem. The alcoholic can not solve their problem until they accept the fact that they are an alcoholic. It is not helpless if one believes in self and your gifts from God. The alcoholic turns to God a lot of the time to help solve their problem. The crucially sick turn to God for a miracle. But it is not the miracle that God gives. He gives acceptance and then the graces to go about and conquer the illness. For the alcoholic, it is the understanding of why they started to drink and the power to fight the urge to drink. For the critically sick, it is hope and blessings to overcome the illness. And for the overweight it is the knowledge to help one lose weight and the courage to fight the craving to over eat.

Losing over one hundred pounds can not be timed. You must give your body whatever time period it needs to lose the weight. Setting your sights on dates can only lead to disappointment if the dates are not met. I know it is a long and hard battle. The ideal of spending one year or longer on a diet is not an easy adjustment. But look at it as a once in a life time adjustment. It is the after effect of all the rewards and good eating that you have done in the pass. Just think about the national debt. Somebody has to pay the money back, whether it is our generation or our children's generation. At some point in time we have to pay the piper. We live in the ninety's, but we are now paying for the greed of the eighty's. Does that make the job of paying the national debt or the greed of the eighty's any easier? Doing what is right is not always pleasant. The truth hurts! Can you find a reason to lose the weight? Can you give up a year or two of your life to diet? Questions that must be answered from the heart. Do not kid yourself, it can only lead to hurt.

The rationale behind not using time frames is that sometimes we set unrealistic dates. We set wish dates. We subconsciously want to end the diet quickly. So we push the target dates to a point where every week we would need a better than average weight loss week. But we can not foresee any of the problems that we may encounter from the diet or from the outside world. Case in point, one day last year, 1994, I was sent home early from work because of a snow storm. As I was driving home I was wondering what I was going to do with all this free time so that I would not eat. With nothing to do, my mind focused on eating to occupy the time. With luck I found something to do, I recorded some tapes that I had put off recording. Before I knew it, the day had passed and I had not eaten anything extra. Later on in my diet I found out why I wanted to eat and hopefully have conquered this problem.

One hundred plus pounds overweight, do what people think can not be done, lose the weight. Prove to yourself that you have what it takes to lose the weight. Do it for self. Do it for the sake of doing it. It will be hard, it will be unbearable at times, but it can be done. Depend on self and not any outside miracles. When all else fails, you can only depend upon yourself and God. Come on, join the club where membership is special and hard to enter. Join the club that many want to enter, but few pass the test. Join the club of people who have lost one hundred plus pounds. It is a membership that you will never forget. I say to you, it can be done. You must will it to be done!!! We all have the mental complexity to conquer our weight problem. The question is can you find the right button to push to start the mind working? Join the club that is low in membership, but eager to have new members. Finally, to you I say find the reason, and the rest is down hill.

The Struggle in the Middle

How much weight do you want to lose? How much weight do you have to lose? This section refers to the people who already have started a diet. But if you are thinking of starting a diet, this may offer you some insight into the struggle in the middle.

Have you ever taken a trip that you just were not totally convinced to do? As you start driving down the highway you just could not wait to get to your destination. Then the mind starts to wonder, what am I going to do once I get there? How are the people going to react? Will I have fun? It is at this point you start to think about turning around and going back home. You realize that it is the same distance back home as to your destination. So you drive onward. It is funny how you forget about the drive once you get to the destination.

The more weight you have to lose, the harder the struggle in the middle. For example, if you want to lose sixty pounds, at the thirty pound range your family and friends start to tell you how good you look. Depending on how hard and how long it takes you to lose weight, you may be more willing to take your current weight lose and quit the diet. If you want to lose ten pounds, then the struggle at the half way point isn't that difficult. Not that it is any easier or harder to lose weight, but you are more focused on your goal. Five pounds is not good enough, you want the whole ten pounds.

What is the struggle in the middle? It is the half way point of any race. It is the minds way of recapping where it has come from. Examining if it can handle where it wants to go. At the halfway point you start to feel better about yourself. You have more energy. You compare your before and after pictures. You feel good about yourself. Some family and friends tell you to stop dieting! That if you lose any more weight you won't look right. The mind may now look for more rewards or start to cheat for a couple of days. If there is no bad after effect from the rewarding or cheating, then one may stop dieting. What makes the half way point so impressive? Is it the fact that it is a milestone? I think that it is a relief. The relief of knowing that you are half way finished. That everything from this point on is downhill. This may be the point where new clothes are needed. The fact that when you walk in the clothing store you are a couple of sizes smaller is a victory in itself.

What makes the middle so special or tough. Its like mid-term in school, this is where you find out how you are doing. Its like spring break, one just wants to forget about studying for a couple days. This helps prepare the mind for finals. The middle struggle is the mid-life review. What have I done to this point? Do I need to improve? Should I relax a little bit more? Can I continue on my current pace? Many questions are asked. Few are answered. It is at this point that I think about the struggle of dieting.

How long does the struggle in the middle last. It can be from a moment to weeks. It can be the moment you step off the scale. Yes, I did it. Nothing can stop me from reaching my goal. Or it can be wow I feel great. Do I really need to continue with this diet? If I just ...., I will lose the rest of the weight with ease. It's like receiving an A on your report card. You know you must keep up the hard work if you expect to get an A on your final report card. The evaluation of the A may take effect now. What did it cost me to get this A. Was it worth the struggle? A grade of B would have been just as nice. Find your mental notch and hold course, because the water can be rough from this point forward.

The struggle in the middle is hardest if one places time frames upon one's self. As in the example with the person who wants to lose sixty pounds, this person will review one key element. How long did it take me to lose thirty pounds? If it took an average of three pounds a week, then it took ten weeks. That is two and a half months. This person now has another two and a half months to go before they reach their goal. Can the mind handle another ten weeks? Ten weeks does not sound like a long time, but the mind now has some information about the day in and day out struggle of dieting. The adjustment the body makes. The counter adjustments the mind has to make. A short term conflict is at hand, do I take a break and prolong the diet process or do I work my way straight to the end? For your family that have not seen you in a couple of months or years, they think you look great. You have done an excellent job losing weight. This is how I felt. The compliment can be overwhelming, but I then realized that I was still overweight. Then my joy had to tamper with the fact that I had a long way to go. Yes, the mind was happy and sad at the same time. The accomplishment was there because I made a milestone. Reality set in knowing I was only half way home.

The struggle in the middle, time to focus on the reason for the diet. The struggle in the middle, no place to drop the anchor. The struggle in the middle, the dull days of the diet.

After the Diet

Everything has a beginning and an ending. There is no difference with a diet. There is usually more emotion at the ending of the diet, then at the beginning of the diet. Successful diets end with joy and happiness. Failed diets end with bewilderment and disappointment. Like many of you, I have had diets end without noticing that the diet was over. Mini diets start and stop without notice. The mind attempts to lose weight without the true effort of dieting.

Once the diet is over, the mind is freed from the restrictions placed upon self. With the successful end of the diet, rewards are now in order. All the food items that were disallowed during the diet are now available. You are now a child in a candy store. Ready to eat whatever your heart desires. For one or two meals this is okay. Now another process has started, how do I keep the weight off? This is a question that is asked, but few want to answer. It is always answered by the dieter, but very rarely is it carried out.

Many times the dieter was aided by a weight maintenance program or an off the shelf diet product. The program and/or products did their job, they helped the dieter lose the weight. This struggle of losing the weight does not help the mind. Once the diet was over, the mind was freed to explore the foods of old. To taste the joys of the past. The mind was a prisoner that was freed from prison, the debt has been paid. But the mind remembers the prison, and does not want to go back to prison! It is this remembrance of the struggle that causes the dieter who gains the weight back not to want to go on another diet. It is like getting one's hand burnt on the kitchen stove when one was a child, one will always be cautious around any stove to ensure one does not get burnt again. It is the first struggle to lose weight that makes any other diet attempt difficult. The dieter becomes gun shy. Doubt surfaces like the sun, always questioning one's ability. Do you think you can do it again? Remembering the pains and struggles of the first diet. Any other diet attempt will always recall past memories of dieting. The failed attempts are the first to flood the mind. The reason to diet is the boat that rolls one to safety.

Can one deduce why they gain the weight back after a successful diet? What did you learn from the diet? Is your reason strong enough to help you keep off the weight? Did the struggle of dieting teach you anything about your eating habits? What is your new relationship with food? So many questions. So few answers. An open mind and heart during a diet leads to an easier transition period after the diet. How you have adapted your diet to fit your life style should help you incorporate these adjustments back into your old life style with some changes. Have a transition plan to handle the after diet eating and exercising. Have the same confidence after the diet to keep the weight off that you had during the diet to take the weight off.

Naturally there will be some after diet adjustments. Your body will adjust to your new eating habits and exercising. This is because as you add different food and change your level of exercise the body will change its level of consumption. The body will burn calories (energy/fuel) at a different level. Also, remember that the amount of food you were eating during the diet was to lose weight. Now you are eating to maintain your current weight. This is a mental adjustment to find the right amount of food that gives you the nutrient value your body needs and the mental satisfaction of eating a good meal.

After diet, weight gains can be the results of emotional needs. The old systems are back on line again, reward, stress management, depression, and joy just to name a few. How you handle these feelings can dictate your weight maintenance program. If you can apply the same rules that helped you during your diet, then you will handle the emotional aspect. Once again, the reason why you dieted in the first place will help you overcome this difficult area.

One must be careful of the senses, taste, smell, and sight. These senses that had to be conquered or controlled during the diet must be controlled after the diet. Taste buds can quickly convert back to the taste buds of before the diet. The temptation from the sight and smell of food can play havoc on the mind. The mind is now free to roam about without any restrictions. What was disallowed is now acceptable. Taste, smell, and sight, do not let them overwhelm you.

The diet is now over! The reason has carried you through the struggles, emotions, and pain of dieting. What was learned about self and food? They said that money can corrupt, so can food, food can corrupt the mind. The dieter has entered another phase, keeping the weight off. The after diet celebration must be tapered with reality. The game is over, but a new game has started. Life is asking you another question, can you keep it off? My response, not a problem!!!

Chapter Seven
The Diet is Working

Compliments

After awhile on your diet you will begin to lose weight. You will notice the weight loss and others will notice the weight loss. It is the compliments on your weight loss that you have to control. Hi, you look good; is always nice to hear. This compliment feeds your reward system. Now you want or deserve a reward. This compliment feeds into your logic, and you begin to question whether or not you need to continue on your diet. A dieter is always looking to end a diet. Sometimes the compliments that we hear gives us the justification to stop dieting. Compliments can turn into questions; 'Why are you on a diet? You look good!' These questions pose a threat when you are questioning your need to continue on your diet. One may use this positive question to end one's diet. The only advice is to remember your reason and your goal. People only see the outside and not the inside. Clothes hide a lot of things. Stick to your original goal, do not let positive compliments hold you back.

Compliments are great but they are one sided. People will tell you when you are losing weight how great you look. They will even ask how you did it. Very, very rarely will people say anything to you when you gain the weight back, not to your face anyway!!!

Compliments should feed your desire to continue on your diet. The struggle is starting to pay off. All the internal hard work is effective. Compliments are external rewards. Compliments give you a chance to take a quick glance at yourself and realize how far you have come. In the same breath it should also give you the courage to continue on. I always like to think of it this way, if you think I look good now, then wait until I'm finished. Compliments are of the present. They represent past work done. You have a mental picture of what you want to look like after the diet. Compare that mental picture to the current you and the previous you, that is the excitement to continue on with the diet.

Remember, compliments do not have to be words, they can be a smile or a nod of the head as people walk by. People are always watching, ready to offer a comment or two, The reason to diet must come from within. Stay strong to your reason and take compliments as a positive re-enforcement to continue on with the struggle. A compliment is a small victory in the battle of the diet. Hi, you look good, keep up the good work!

Outward Appearance

What goes on behind closed doors may be totally different then what is seen. The outward appearance may not show the struggles of dieting. Your outward look, behind clothes, does not show your problem areas that keep you dieting. Dieting is a one on one battle with self. No one truly knows another's struggle with dieting. Words of encouragement can offer comfort. But words sometimes do not offer relief. All is calm to the world, but the struggle is intense within the walls of the mind. This is every dieter's challenge. Just like a baby will tense with the coming of teeth, so too at some point, will a dieter struggle with their diet. As the baby sleeps in peace, a mother knows the pain of the baby. Unlike the baby, only the dieter truly understands their struggle.

Outward appearance is that the diet is going well. Compliments flow as freely as rain from the sky. Only the clouds know how much more rain they contain. Only the clouds know when it will stop. Man can only predict the weather. So too will people predict whether on not you continue with your diet. They constantly look for you to slip, to fall. This judgment is made on past failed diets by them or a friend or a family member. Man will look at a cloud and say it will rain. Man will look at an overweight person and say that person will not lose weight. It is from past history that this judgment is made. More often than not, man is right about the overweight person and wrong about the weather. Is it the outward appearance that judges us or is it history? One must learn from history. Find a strong reason and history will not repeat itself.

Outward appearance of a person on a diet, is like a person in quick sand, will the person sink or reach safety? The quick sand is the mind, constantly struggling to free itself from the diet. The person sinks when they give in to the quick sand, the weight. They sink because they panic. They move without cause, constantly changing direction, and finally giving up. The person reaches safety by understanding the situation. Searching for tools to pull them to safety. Conserving energy so as not to anger the quick sand. Slow moving toward land to grab the tree branch or rope to pull them to safety. Outwardly the world sees a person in quick sand and says, the quick sand has acquired another person.

Outwardly the world is slow to praise, but quick to criticize. Outwardly the world is quick to tell one to lose weight, but fails to tell you how to lose weight. Outward appearance and dieting, does anyone truly understand your struggle? Pass or fail, the more you are overweight, the more you are judged to fail. Take the challenge, find a reason and outwardly prove the world they are wrong about you. Do not judge me like everyone else, it may take some time, but I will overcome!!!

Chapter Eight
The Review of Self

Time Frame, Can You Really Judge It

One of the most complex things in this universe is the human body. Of the human body, the mind must be the most complicated. Just think for a moment, how the body fights off germs. How the body protects itself from adverse conditions. Even how the body stores energy for later consumption. The way the body sends signals back and forth to the brain. The brain constantly sending signals to the heart to pump blood to the body. Is the body only doing what is natural, or is the brain hard at work making key decisions, even while we sleep? So complex is the brain / mind, that even in deep sleep, in the state of a dream, the body can send signals to the brain to interrupt a dream because the body needs some type of relief, be it the need to go to the bathroom or a glass of water. Yet with all this information, one can not control ones weight reduction process. If the brain controls the body, then why cannot I tell my body not to store any extra food today, that anything it does not need, to treat as waste? Do the muscles act independent of the brain? Does the left side of the brain know what the right side is doing? Or has technology evolved faster than our instinct for eating?

Let's examine the caveman. They hunt for their food. Food had to be consumed when it was killed or it would spoil. So the time between meals could last for days. Then, over time man moved along the technology scale to the point where he could grow, raise (cattle and poultry), catch (fish) his food. Men and woman who worked in the fields and/or on ships, more than made up for any overeating they may have done. Once again the body's defenses saved and used the energy from the food wisely. Here we are today, wondering why the body saves all this energy. Why doesn't the body just disregard its extra food? Why cannot I enjoy all the food I want without paying the price by gaining weight? Why does the body keep the extra food while the mind knows it doesn't need the energy?

The body has protection mechanisms independent of the mind. Have you ever wondered how people can go on hunger strikes without losing too much weight? The body's or more notably, the muscle groups have ways of anticipating when extra energy will be needed and can prepare for it. An example is weight training with different level of weights. If one is going to do three reps of an exercise with three different pounds of weights, one does not increase the weights in straight increments. That is, you do not go from 20 pounds to 30 pounds to 40 pounds. This is, because the muscle expects the next increase and prepares for the increase. To maximum the exercise, the mind must trick the muscle by varying the weights. That is, you could start at 20 pounds then go to 40 pounds followed by 30 pounds, or start at 30 pounds, then increase to 40 pounds and finish off with 20 pounds. Notice how the mind and body work independent of each other?

So I ask you, can you judge your time frame to lose weight? Can you say I will lose ten pound in a month without truly understanding your body? Can you say that I will lose four inches off my waist in two month when you do not understand how your body stores the fat cells? Time frames should not be written in stone!!!

I'm not saying that one should not set goals. But sometimes we live by our goals and if we do not meet these goals we get disappointed and agitated. Our diet starts to lose its purpose

76

and we start to convince ourselves that we will never lose weight. Yes, we begin to challenge our reason for going on the diet. Time frame and goals will most likely be met with regularity in the beginning weeks of a diet. It is after the body has time to adjust to the changes that are being made that cause time frames to be hard to judge. It will take days to weeks before the body believes that this reduced food consumption is constant and reacts by reducing energy used.

Take for an example some of the advertising techniques used by the weight reduction programs. They promise that in a couple of weeks you can lose ten to fifteen pounds. Even some of the exercise manufacturers state that in the first 30 days you can lose ten to twenty pounds. They do not make these kind of statements over a longer period of time because they understand how the body adjusts to reduce food consumption or an exercise program. It is the fat burning process that is so difficult to judge. Some people burn a higher percentage of fat than others.

So much information is needed to make good judgment about setting goals for reducing weight over time. It is not always wise to judge by one means if a diet is processing effectively. For an example, I was judging my diet by the scale. I was looking for an average of three pound a week. For one whole month during the middle of my diet, I did not lose one pound. For four weeks it was very disappointing. Wondering if I would ever reach my goal. But what I noticed was that during that month, some how, some way, I lost two inches off my waist. It was at that point that I had to realign my thinking about measuring the progress of my diet. Before this time, I never gave thought to the fact that people could tell I was losing weight by looking at my face. I realized that I could not tell simply because I was always looking at my face and since the reduction is always small, I adjusted to the new features of my face.

Another explanation why I say it is hard to judge your time frame is that once you start an exercise program, a transformation takes place in your body. The fat cells are replaced with muscle, and muscle cells weigh more than fat cells. So, it will take you time to adjust your level of thinking and understanding what is going on in your body. It is hard enough with simple food reduction to judge an accurate time schedule for your diet, adding simple exercise, like walking, jogging, or riding a stationary bike, is a little more difficult to judge. Adding weight training to the process makes it that much harder.

Finally, one of the last explanations why it is hard to judge a time schedule for weight reduction is that it varies by weight categories. Your body adjusts the amount of calories it needs to burn daily. That means, you have to work harder to maintain the same weekly weight loss. An example, at 250 pounds if I ate 2000 calories per day I will lose two to three pounds during that week. At 210 pounds if I ate 2000 calories per day I would only lose one to two pounds per week. The same holds true for exercise. The more your weigh, the more calories you will burn during an exercise session. So, to hold the same level of weight loss during an entire diet period without changes to the level of consumption can only lead to disappointment at some point in time.

The more you understand your body and how it reacts to food and/or exercise the better you will feel mentally about your diet and your progress. Take in mind when you set your weight loss goals, the unexpected. The night out with the boys or girls, the holidays, and the need to cheat (DCD). Good luck in setting your weight target and time frame. Choose logically and remember, judge not by others but by self! What's good for the Jones' may not be good for you. Be individual! This is not a race with anyone, but yourself. So you cannot win and you cannot lose to yourself. If you need longer to reach your goal, then do not let your time frame hold you back. See you at the finish line!!!

The Quote,
"The Easiest Person to Deceive is Oneself"

Adults hold back the words. Their words are sugar coated with nicety. They speak the truth behind your back. Children, especially the very young, speak the truth. They say their true feelings. Their words echo truth, they send you searching for comfort from within yourself. Yes, the words of a little girl, 'Mommy, he is fat!' Those words hurt more than the same words from anyone else. Your doctor can echo the same words, but they do not have the same feeling. Family and friends can say it with the same intensity, but you can defend against them, they love you anyway. But there are no answers to the young one's statement. The hard cold truth sends you reeling for comfort, the refrigerator.

The young do not only speak the truth to adults, but to other children as well. They tease the heavy set kids. Calling them porky pig, elephant, and fat boy or fat girl among other things. They, the heavy set children, get excluded out of most of the games, but they adjust to this fact. For some, it makes them stronger, for others they fall prey and never fully recover from this for the rest of their lives. Still some look upon it as an unhappy childhood. For a few of the heavy set kids, they grow out of it, it was family genes that made them heavy.

Deep down in the core of your memory are built in excuses why you cannot lose weight. The real truth is that the reason was never good enough. The mind could not motivate the will to fight. So we fall back to what is comfortable, food. The statement holds truth, 'The easiest person to deceive is oneself." Why, because you know your strengths and weakness. So you tell yourself what you want to hear and believe, and hold back all other information. A criminal never believes they will get caught, even if the police have caught everyone who committed a crime.

The child spoke the truth. The hurt only lasts for a moment. The pleasure of a good meal lasts longer. The hurt of the truth is overcome by the comfort of the food. But what makes the words of the young child hurt even more, is that it was spoken in the house of GOD. At that point there is no defense. One simply acknowledges that fact. For a moment one begins to move forward, to start to search for a reason. But as the child leaves ones line of sight and space of hearing, the thoughts quickly fade. Like anything else, this is a perfect place to start the search for a reason. Ask for help from God and you shall receive. Be alert, because what you may receive is not the actual weight loss, but a reason to lose the weight, and that's half of the battle.

Lessons can be learned from war. Before World War II started, England and France could have stopped Germany from invading another country. But England and France did not have the will to fight, so they gave in to Germany's demands. Unfortunately, England and France's signals of weakness give Germany the upper hand. In the end, England and France had no choice but to fight or lose control of their counties to Germany. If England or France had the will to fight in the beginning, millions of people would not have died. The lesson from all of this is that until the reason is strong enough for the struggle, the body will suffer, and it will take longer to lose the weight. It may even cost you total victory.

An example of deceiving oneself and a lesson from World War II. At twenty pounds overweight, one does not think one is fat. A little stomach may be contributed to the beer or wine one drinks. So at this point one just keeps going with their normal habits. At thirty to fifty pounds overweight, one may begin to feel overweight, but your friends start to call you big guy or the new sports' term wide body. So you feel comfortable with that. Some may even call it love fat. The mind begins it's defensive process by saying that it can lose the weight anytime it wants. At fifty to seventy pounds overweight the need to lose weight is now more of

80

a concern. The friendly names your friends still call you, offer you no more comfort as it did before. You begin to change some of your habits hoping to lose a few pounds. At first you succeed in losing some weight, but you added those few pounds you lost plus a few more pounds. At this point you may start some of the diet programs to help you lose some weight. But deep down you still think that when you're ready, you will lose the weight. Now with the summer gone and with winter's cold spells settling in, old habit quickly come back. Now you are in the seventy to one hundred pound overweight range. Denial starts to set in. I can not believe I'm this big. You add some nice clothes to your wardrobe and you start to feel good about yourself again. You still do the same thing about dieting you do in the fifty to seventy pounds range, but this time you try a little harder. With luck you will not go any higher in weight gain. But luck was not on your side. You are now one hundred plus pounds overweight. If you were not at war before with your weight, you are now. You start to look at all the ads in the newspapers and magazines. You start to try a few magic weight loss programs with mixed results. After a certain point you give in to the weight. Your thought process now accepts the fact that you will be overweight the rest of your life. Still you try more programs, with the same mixed results.

What are you searching for? The same thing England and France did during W.W.II, a powerful ally. With this powerful ally and your own will to win, the fight is long and hard, but after one or two years you did it, you lost the weight. But what did it take to do it? A reason to fight. The will to fight through the struggle, and your ability to find within you what you needed to help you win. For England and France it was a powerful ally, for you it my be a loved one to give you encouragement. Remember two things happened, one, you stopped deceiving yourself, and two, you found a reason.

The mind will always defend itself. Most people do not like to have their logic questioned. Are we telling ourselves the truth about our weight problem, or are we too weak to face the struggle to lose the weight? Do we have that belief that the world has placed upon us, after a certain weight one needs help to effectively lose weight? If there is a problem deep within your mind about your weight, you will not lose the weight until that problem is solved. Temporary loss yes, permanent loss no.

Understanding Self

The search for a reason must come from within. The most understood person you know is yourself. The least understood person you know is yourself. All diets fail or succeed in this area. Diets either come from within or they are excuses. A diet may be nothing more that a temporary excuse to get family and friends off you back about losing weight. A diet may be nothing more than an excuse to oneself that one can not lose weight and justifies the constant eating. It is this understanding in the beginning that must be conquered. It is the search for reason, a motivating factor that must be found. It is the preparation of the will to succeed that must be re-enforced. Everyone has it within themselves. The question is, how long can the light burn? How long can you keep yourself motived? The game is four quarters, three sets, or eighteen holes long. Can you survive the game without burning out in the first half? Can you motive yourself or do you need help? Self wants to lose weight. Self wants the self of yesteryear. Self wants, but self is not worth the struggle. It is the long struggle that self does not want to go through. It is not that self can not do the struggle, but the reason is not there. Once again the 'Why' question is asked. Self still does not have an answer. The search for a reason, how can I motive myself?

It is time to do some soul searching. It is time to look past our own internal defenses. It is time to ask ourselves some hard questions. But this time we must come back with the true answers. Not the answers we give to the world, not the cover-up, but the underline reason. Our weight problem may be caused by some other problem that we have. Our unwillingness to say no to a friend when asked to go out and have a couple of drinks. Eating to aid our depression. Eating as a stress relief. Eating because of happiness. Eating for comfort. Maybe we hide behind our weight. Using the weight to justify other aspects of our life. Using weight as the excuse. It is in understanding that one gains wisdom. It is wisdom that gives one courage. It is courage that causes one to fight. It is in fighting that we overcome the enemy. Diplomacy does not work when it comes to losing weight. The body does not have the ability. The body only knows survival. It is this natural need to survive that keeps the extra weight. It is the mind that must fight. It is a battle of wants versus needs. The body's needs versus the mind's wants. It is this understanding that can be learned during the diet process. It is during the struggling that intelligence about oneself is gained.

Life is a challenge. Life is a constant learning process. Continually changing and evolving. God asks the questions, can you change? Can you be more compassionate to your neighbor? Work asks the question, can you improve on the current product or system? Can you think of a way to improve quality and perform your job faster and cheaper? Your children challenge you with their willingness to learn. Yet, it is the challenge to self that is hardest to accept. It is the uncertain water ahead that trouble us. It is life on a diet. It is self denial. We have changed many avenues of our life because we do not want to be denied. We surround ourselves by friends and people who tells us what we want to hear. They re-enforce the negative images that we have about ourselves. Very few friends are willing to tell the truth. It happens in many relationships. It is only when there is no other recourse that the truth is told. We walk with blinders on our minds. But what does this have to do about dieting? Have you ever examined why a diet failed? Can you point to one thing that caused your slip? Is it the need for relief, stress management? Is it the self denial and the craving for non diet food? Is it not understanding your own needs, both mentally and physically? Is it the non belief in the reason for dieting?

Dieting is an art. The people who master the arts have a good understanding of themselves. They have the ability to overcome their weakness. They turn a negative into a positive. They learn from their mistakes. We all do this in some area of our lives. Can we transform this to dieting? The strong willed will fight to overcome the struggle of dieting. Others look for outside help, which may never arrive. The mind wants help, but does not know how to go about getting help. Can we all lose weight? Yes, but self must be willing to fight. The fighting is an art. The true art of dieting is to diet without dieting. To simply make changes that are mentally acceptable. To say I do not want this cake today because I do not need the cake. Self must challenge self. Self must motive self. Self must defend self.

Understanding self is a defensive measure. During a diet if one is open to oneself, one will learn one's weakness. It is learning that certain situations one just can not handle during the diet process. It may be eating out, going to parties, or simply having desserts in the house. It is the temptation that these things pose to the mind that is hard to handle. It is amazing how self denial can lead to craving, craving of something under other situations you would not want. Self denial challenges the mind. Self denial questions the logic behind the NO answer. Self denial temps with, who's going to know you have cheated? Self denial is especially working if you join a weight loss center. Self denial, it's the good versus bad. Self denial, it started with Adam and Eve. From man's beginning we have been questioning ourselves. Always asking why, but for the dieter the answer must be the reason.

Understanding self is being true to self. The first step is to accept failure. To diet one can not be scared to fail. To cheat does not mean self does not have the will power. To cheat is a self break. It takes courage to know that from time to time one needs a break from dieting. To cheat means to accept that one is human. It is the understanding of knowing when a break is needed so that it can be planned. Self denial can burn down the internal systems. Self denial must be understood just like one must learn the body's telling signals. Just like the body gives signals when it is thirsty or hungry, so to will the mind when it needs a break from the diet. It is over time that one learns the signals, but to succeed one must know that there will be signals. All of life is signals, be it from God above down to the earth we stand on. There is always a warning of danger. It is a learning process to recognize the warnings. To understand what is being stated. Do not deny self beyond your critical point, but do not give into self either. The reason constantly defines the critical point. The stronger the reason, the greater the desire. The greater the desire the lower the critical point.

Understand the game that has engulfed self. Understand that not only is self trying to understand the adjustment being performed by the body, but self has outside forces at work. Self is being attack by friend and foe. No longer is there comfort within the mind. Now the mind is in its own battle. Dieting asks, can you pick up your cross? The cross says, it will not be easy, but it is worth the struggle. It is a challenge just to look at the cross with an open mind and heart. Dieting is a look inward at self without realizing. Dieting is just one more challenge of life.

Self now ponders who am I. Self now begins to question, why me? Self now doubts if the task of dieting is greater than self's ability? But just then from deep within comes the will to succeed. The confidence to achieve. The reason to struggle. The USA found it in the GULF war. What is it? It is a quality that can not be explained. It is a feeling. It can not be tasted. It can not be seen. It can not be heard. But like fear, it can be sensed; confidence in one's abilities. Doubt no longer. Question no more. Believe it can be done and it will. Do not accept no for an answer. Do not let self down. Everybody else lets self down, your teachers, your friends, your employer, your family, and even your parents, but don't let self fail self. Self will find a way to win. Don't let self down. The reason is within. Self is the reason. To say self is not worth the struggle is to give up on life. To say temporary self denial of dieting is not worth the struggle is to say one is an addict to fatty foods. Do not let self down!!! Ponder no more, the word has been given. The cross is you!

Faith Approach

Faith is a wonderful thing to have. We each have our own belief in God. We have a country that was built on this faith. So to must a dieter have faith. Faith does not mean that we do not have to do anything, it means the opposite. It means that during the struggle of life we will receive help when we need it the most.

The dieter must have belief in their self. The reason for dieting must come from within. The reason must come from the heart. When the reason comes from the heart, then it is truly something that we want. It is at this point that faith comes into play. There are times during the diet process that we are weak, that we just do not have the will to fight on. Self has become the struggle, but self does not want to quit, to cheat. It is at this moment that one must rely on faith. It is at this point when one should seek help from God. I'm not trying to force religion on you. If you do not believe, then seek the help of a close friend or someone special. When self can not temporarily handle the struggle of dieting, then self must find an outside source that is worth the struggle. Someone or something that can give you that moment of courage to fight the temptation or craving. It is this underlining faith that must surface. Faith in God and faith in self, that any mountain placed in your path can be climbed or overcome.

Faith is an ideal, a belief. Faith is greatest when we are in trouble or in doubt. Why should we not use the same faith approach to dieting? Dieting is just another one of life struggles. We all have a tendency to sit back and ask God why me? What have I done wrong to deserve this treatment? But we fail to ask the next question; how do I get out of this situation. When the answer arrives, we most of the time either do not believe the answer or are too weak hearted to execute the solution. It is at this moment that faith is weak.

Faith may not be a miracle. Faith is small, small as a mustard seed. Faith is in doing, in confronting the problem. Faith is doing what is right no matter what the cost. Dieting is eating right and exercising. Dieters make hard choices everyday. Eating right is not always fun and it has a cost to the mind, depression. But faith and dieting have a common ground, it is the results. A dieter needs faith, faith in one's self. A dieter also needs faith in outside sources, the good outside sources help the dieter adhere to their diet. The bad outside sources tempt the dieter to cheat. There are the neutral outsides sources, they make the dieter help themselves, and then there is God supplying the inspiration to be good. Dieting is a mental challenge of doing what is right, what is needed versus what is wanted. So many things are done out of want, that it can lead one astray.

Faith is knowing that at every step of the diet process there is help and assistance. Faith is knowing that the answer is within the walls of your heart. Faith is a desire to do what is right, no matter what the cost. Faith is the underlying thing in all of us. Can you muster that faith to help you diet? Trust and faith is within the mind. Every dieter must have faith, at least with themselves, to overcome the struggles of dieting. See you at the finish line, I have faith.

Chapter Nine
Ending Thoughts

Reasons to diet surface like day changing to night. Yet not one of the reasons is good enough for the struggle. Many have tried to diet. Many have succeeded in their diet only to see the weight come back. Yet there is still a desire to diet, but not the courage. Each new day brings another reason to diet and every night brings a cause not to diet. Shallow reasons drown in the struggles of dieting. Shallow reasons are quick answers to a complex problem. Shallow reasons justifies failure. Shallow reasons are the trap of the want and reward systems. Deep within the cobwebs of the mind is a reason to diet. This reason is greater then the struggle to diet, but to find this reason takes time, commitment, and truthfulness. This reason digs up old problems that need to be conquered. This reason gives relief to the pains of dieting. This reason comforts you in your moment of uncertainty or discomfort. This reason gives you your daily bread to survive during this period of dieting. This reason aids you in your time of need. This reason is a teddy bear for a child, a cane for an old person, a job for the family bread winner. The reason is whatever you need to get through the day. The reason, a battle cry to action!!!

Dieting is no different then any other struggle in life, it takes commitment. Dieting is an internal battle to overcome self's defenses. Dieting encompasses so many things and emotions, simply because food has such great importance to the mind and body. It takes a good reason to be able to deny self the foods that self has become accustom to eating. But with the right reason there is no stopping you. The reason is why the war is worth fighting.

In this book I tried to give you some insight into the hidden struggles of dieting. To explain some of the feelings and issues that often go unnoticed. These issues go unnoticed because our subconscious handles these issues. We fail to put the pieces together of failed diets because many of the pieces are who we are. Bad habits are learned and very hard to remove. Sometimes we do not know we have the bad habits. Dieting and food are at opposite ends of the spectrum. Food brings happiness. Dieting brings discomfort and sadness. Food is all around us. We are confronted by food from morning to dust. Dieting implies commitment and disciple. Dieting is a subset of life. Life almost comes to a stop for the one who diets. It is these challenges of life that confronts the dieter and causes many dieters to re-think their commitment to their diet. But the commitment to overcome the challenges of life on a diet is needed. Self is always worth the struggle. When one knows how, there is always a way around the difficulties.

I hope this book has opened your thinking cap and challenged you to address what is holding you back from meeting your weight loss goals. Unlike some others, I have gone through the struggles of dieting. These challenges have changed me, and some of my family and friends. It is not easy to tell someone they need to lose weight without giving them some options on how to lose weight. I have learned a lot about myself in this diet process because I was open minded. I accepted the fact that I did not have the answer, but I knew the answer I needed was out there. Most of all I was determine not to let myself down. I was going to do what so many of my family and friends though could not be done!!! For you see, I was what they called obese. I was One Hundred and Fifty Eight pounds overweight. My model during my diet was no excuses!!! The moment you find one excuse, then you open a flood gate. Once I started walking during my diet, I would walk in the rain, sleet, or snow. The weather did not matter, I was determine to succeed. For me, my reason was worth the struggle. My reason started with the fact that my doctor told me that I needed to lose thirty pounds before he could operate on my knee. He told my that I could not play any basketball, football, or baseball. That if I played any active sports, I would probably need a knee cap replacement in a couple of years. With this reason, I set course on my diet. I wanted to be able to play sports again. The idea of not playing basketball, football, or baseball again was unthinkable. After seven months and seventy pounds, my doctor told me I no longer needed the knee operation. That by losing the weight I relieved the pressure off my knee. With this news I was feeling great. But the doctor asked me a question that I did not give a second though to, Are you going to stay on your diet? I answered yes to his question. For deep down I had found my true reason to diet. You see, getting overweight, I broke a promise I made to myself when I was overweight before. The promise that I made to myself was that I was not going to get overweight again. By getting overweight again, I let myself down. This I would not allow to happen again, but first I had to lose the weight which I had gained. My reason was simple, I did not want to let self down.

In the end it is up to you to find it within yourself to succeed on your diet. There are books available on various methods to diet. But the simplest thing to do without the added expense is to exercise, watch what you eat, and cut the fat out of your diet. That is the easy part, doing it is the hard part. Find the **reason** and you will succeed. Good Luck and God bless!!!